BEAUTIFUL YOGA FOR CHILDREN

Written By Katrina Grimmett
Photography by Andy Pattenden Photography
Copyright@2023 by Kat Grimmett

INTRODUCTION

Yoga and meditation to me is like a breath of fresh air, with the sun warming your skin and feeling awash with peaceful, calm, loving energy within. When I became a mum to my daughter Bella, I wanted to share my love of yoga with her. I wanted Yoga to be an example of how having a daily practise in ones life can gift you with a stable ground to stand upon each day, and offers calm from the busy sensory world we are exposed to. Yoga gently takes one by the hand, turns us inwards to experience love and contentment.

Sparkle Yoga, a children's yoga class was born in 2018 and so far so good, Bella still attends the classes. Bella has been my greatest teacher in showing me how to create a fun and connecting class and I regularly run the lesson plans by her for her opinion. I have received her input for ideas, games and themes on many occasions!

This book is our journey together in designing and practising years of children's yoga classes which engage children, connecting them with the seasons, nature and wildlife. Classes that open hearts to others by learning about different beliefs and ways of life. And, that provides children space to connect with themselves to experience their inner peace and calm.

I hope that as a parent, or teacher, that these classes may bring you confidence in delivering Yoga to children and also bring your community as much joy, love, laughter and connection as we have experienced.

Namaste

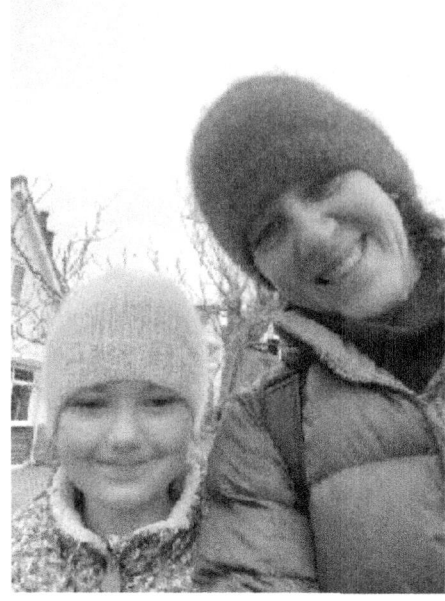

GETTING STARTED

Getting qualified. There are many children's yoga teacher training courses out there and it really is a necessity to take a specific yoga teacher training and certification in children's yoga. Such a course will teach you how to structure and manage children's yoga classes which are very different to an adult yoga class. With an overwhelming amount of programs out there theres a lot to consider when choosing a course.

To help research a course thats right for you, you may want to consider whether you want to take a live or online Yoga teacher training course. An online course allows you to work at your own pace and potentially a more affordable option. An in person course gives the opportunity to interact with a teacher for support. Many online courses also offer this option.

Its a good idea to research the prerequisites required for any course, some companies have no prerequisites others may require you to be a qualified Yoga teacher. Research the cost of the course and compare it with other similar courses. Its a big investment for you and finding one that fits your budget whilst offering you good value for money, continued support and a proven way to teach successful children's yoga classes is advisable.

USEFUL EQUIPMENT

The most essential item needed for a class are yoga mats for each child, preferably sticky mats. A selection of mats in a variety of colours brings a bright fresh and cheerful feel to a room. There are different ways to set up a yoga room using the mats, an example of a set up that is positive and welcoming to the children is to place a rainbow coloured parachute in the middle of the room and then arrange the yoga mats around the parachute, this circular environment brings a positive energy where everyone is included. When buying bulk don't forget to check out companies that offer trade discounts to yoga teachers.

Setting up the room ready for the yoga class is important and taking into consideration the light, temperature, and comfort of it will help a successful session. Breathing exercises may require a window to be open for some fresh air to be circulated. Having cushions may help the comfort for children when sitting.

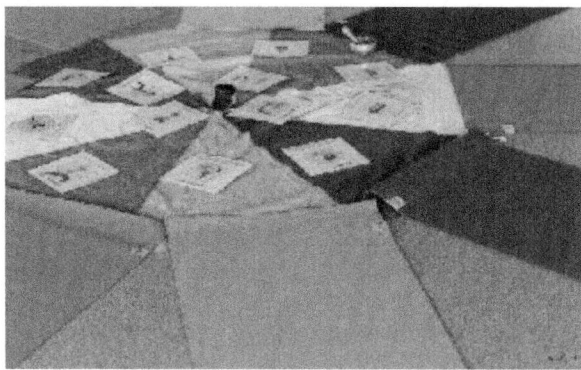

Having a theme and a selection of props available will help enrich the classes. Below are some suggestions for props for children's yoga classes.

Yoga cards with pictures and names of children's yoga postures is a perfect addition to any children's yoga class. They can offer children an empowering choice of choosing postures that they like, they can also be used in so many different ways for games and activities. Purchasing the right cards for you may take a bit of research to see which ones you like.

As the children become more experienced and older in age, creating some more challenging yoga pose cards is a good idea, this offers progression and challenges for the children as they develop in their yoga practise.

Having a props basket set up for the class can inspire the children and yourself to be spontaneous with ideas of new poses and games for example. Colourful muslins is a wonderful prop that can be used in many imaginative ways, like using as wings of an animal or a super hero cape. These sorts of props can also be used whilst in poses, for example, floating the material up and down using arms, or for relaxation as a blanket, or to watch the end of the material being moved to help concentration.

Colourful bean bags is another excellent prop that can be used to help in balance poses, and also as an inspiring prop for games. Having colourful props is an excellent way to engage children through play and visual appeal.

Having musical instruments, like chimes or a Tibetan Singing Bowl is a great way to get attention or to change an activity. Sound can also be used to help children focus during a relaxation. Having equipment that can play music can be helpful for background sounds, for playing games, relaxation, or even for guided meditation.

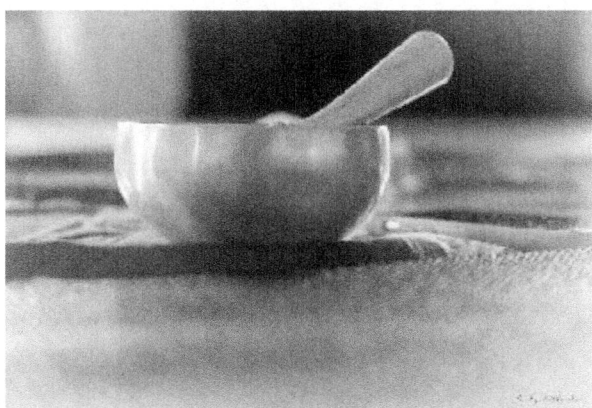

A box of small hand held instruments such as shakers, drums and bells are a fun addition to bring to the classes. Such instruments can offer children opportunities for enhancing their listening, concentration and team working skills. Creating a musical masterpiece together is a really fun activity.

It is important for an instructor to feel and show excitement about the props and introduce them to the children. There are many more creative props an instructor can bring and endless ways in which the imagination can use them, for example, wooden animals, skipping ropes, cones, yoga bricks, ribbons, balls and balloons.

Props for creative use is also another inspiring thing to bring to a class. Story books, puppets, pens, paper, crayons, paint, scissors, fabrics, wool and much more can be used. Having a theme or learning objective can help give choice of what to bring to help inspire the children's imagination and learning experience. Paint pens are a great choice for paint offering minimal mess and minimal waste, they also last well. Purchasing or collecting non toxic materials and natural materials fits well with the philosophy of yoga, in respecting and caring for nature and the world around us. Other suggestions for craft materials that have been successful in classes are natural feathers, rocks, shells, sticks, wool or cotton, wooden beads and paper.

Reading books to the children is a beautiful enhancement to any yoga class. Books can be used to theme a class around or stories can be read at the end of the class that connects with the theme whilst the children engage in a craft activity. Short story books provide variety for selection and are cost effective. Stories from around the World, that follow a year, or about animals are some suggested book themes to have and can also be used time and time again.

YOGA TEACHER QUALITIES

A yoga teacher should be an example of a person living a yogic life. One of having their own practise, knowledge of asanas, mindfulness and acting with presence and compassion. A children's yoga teacher needs to be enthusiastic, friendly, and understanding of children. A leader needs to create an atmosphere where children are free and are encouraged to express themselves.

A children's yoga teacher should be clear, calm and confident when giving instruction. To help with this an instructor may want to start with simpler asanas and activities and then begin to incorporate more challenging ones as they and the children gain experience and confidence together. Being present with children during a class will help in connecting with the children and in meeting their energy and needs.

Giving positive feedback to the children during a class is really important in helping to build the children's confidence and self-esteem. If a child is safe and having fun in a pose then there is no need to continually correct them, as this could be detrimental to their self-confidence. Giving specific feedback, rather than just a well done, will be more meaningful to the children.

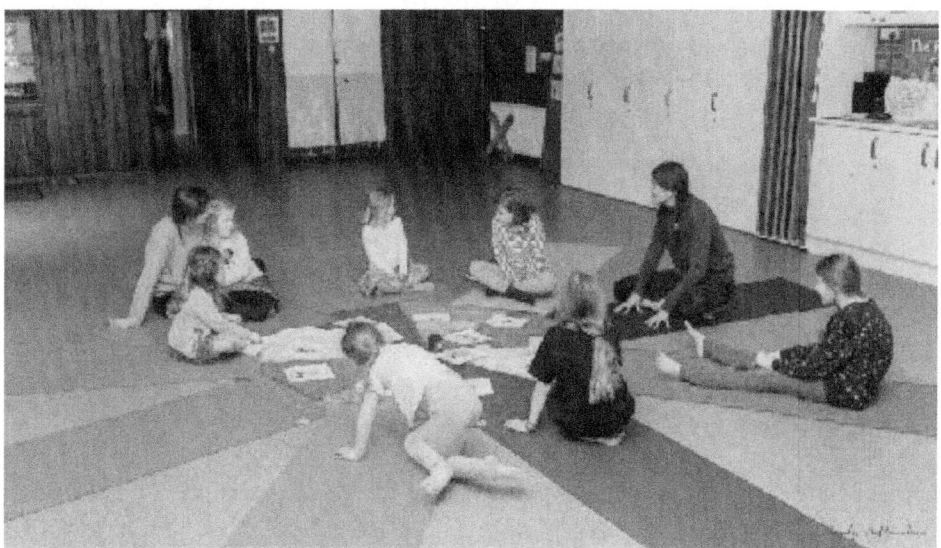

GUIDELINES FOR CLASSES

Some guidelines are needed for a class to run successfully. Being respectful to each other and the environment is an all-encompassing quality for all for a class to function well.

There will be occasions when children are restless or fidgety for many possible reasons, hunger, worries in their lives outside of the class, not able to concentrate, among many other reasons. This is very normal for children and an instructor could try to meet these energy shifts with spontaneous ideas, for example, a short drink break or a change of activity.

At times children need to do something different than asked, or they are unable to concentrate. It is ok for a child to be free to not do something asked or to not join in with a pose or activity being done, but what is important is the respect of others whilst they wish to do something else.

A quiet area could be a good suggestion for an instructor to have when children are not wishing to join in or do something the rest of the class is doing. The quiet area could offer a mindful activity such as colouring in a mandala. This gives a child an opportunity to be still and to reconnect with themselves and allows them time to try to work out what they need to do to refocus their energy to enjoy the rest of the class.

A child may need more support and an instructor, when able may want to try to connect further with any children, creating a patient and safe environment for them to express their feelings.

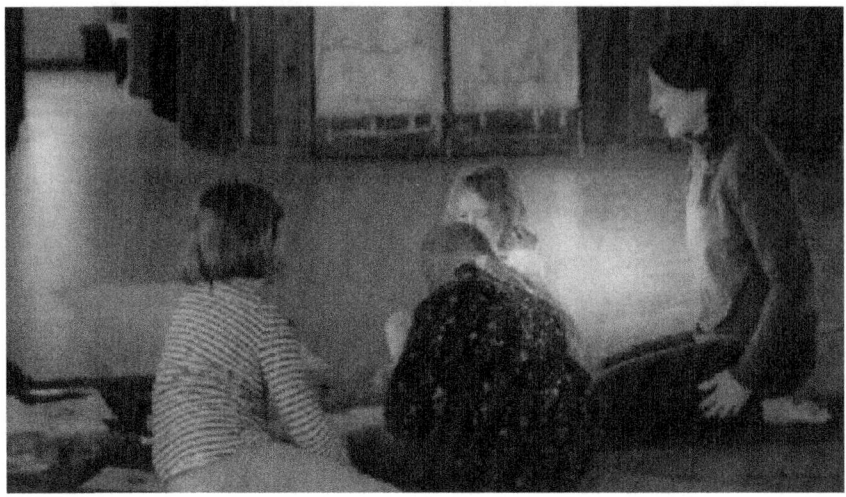

THE CHILDREN

Children need to feel physically comfortable during a yoga class. No specific clothing is required, however wearing certain types of clothing can be beneficial. Good fitting leggings and leotards work really well, or clothing that is flexible and that allows the body to move freely. Tracksuit bottoms with t-shirts tucked in is another good choice. Fabrics that have breathable abilities and that are designed to wick away moisture is beneficial to keep the user feeling cool and dry, but not necessary.

Assessing the children's ages, interests, and attention span, needs to be considered when planning a class. It is believed and supported with theory, that age of a child doesn't always give accurate information about their experience, interests, strengths and abilities and individual children will develop at different stages. It is important to consider every child attending the session and meet them at their level of experience, interests and skills to ensure that every child's needs are met.

CHILDREN AGED 3-5 YEARS

Children aged 3 to 5 years old are full of fun, they are fast, full of energy and their imaginations can run wild. Children of this age group love playing and moving and a yoga class will need to be made active to meet this energy. It is hard for children of this age group to sit still or stay in one pose for a long time. A yoga instructor teaching this age group will need to let each pose and game flow and to not hesitate for too long between activities. If the children are allowed to release their energy through games and poses, they then should be able to lie at the end of a class and practise imaginary relaxation.

They are physically active and their physical ability enables them to now, run and stop, jump, hop, stand on one leg and use facial expressions. They have become much more coordinated with running. They can catch a ball easily and able to kick a ball forward. They are so active, and may even use actions for words, for example, they may run around with their arms out wide rather than say the word, aeroplane. Their left or right hand is now established. Their ability to concentrate in controlling their hands are more established and they are able to copy a circle or pick up small blocks and build a tower.

Active play is critical for their development. Yoga poses and active games can help children to develop their coordination, balance, gross motor skill and fine motor skills. Active children tend to be leaner and healthier and less likely to be inactive in adulthood. Helping children to use up their natural energy also promotes better eating and sleeping habits.

A child's body of this age is also changing, their shape more than height and weight develops. Their bones in the skull and face are growing, their shoulders begin to narrow and their posture improves, the toddler tummy now flattens.

This is a great age for crafts and the practise of cutting, painting, colouring and crafting should be enjoyable. Self help skills are also developing, like feeding and dressing themselves.

Yoga poses and games should involve movements that develop a child's body awareness and that are easily explained. The exercises should be short and lively to help maintain their energy and concentration.

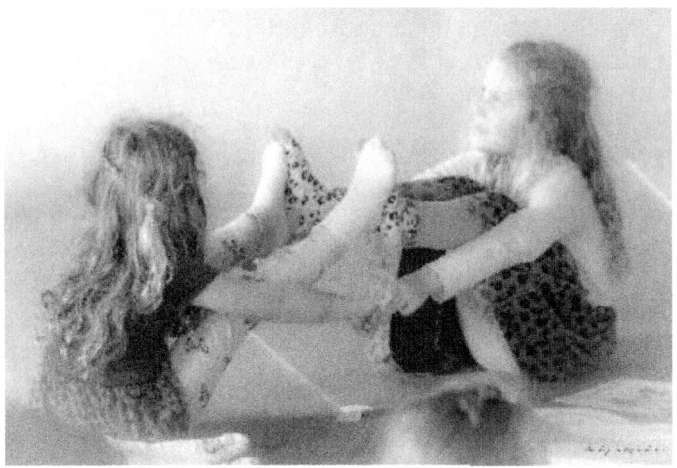

This age group do have great powers of imagination. Playing allows children time to truly let their imaginations run wild and create worlds of their own that they have control over. They love to create imaginary worlds, characters and plots, these can also sometimes match their emotional state. Imaginary play can help them to learn to express and regulate their feelings. Through this type of play children can learn to cope with their emotions as they act our fear, frustration and anger in a situation that they can control. It is also a chance for them to practise empathy and understanding.

Imaginary play can also give children a sense of accomplishment and satisfaction, and can help build their confidence and self perception. Playing with other children is cooperative play helps children develop their social skills as they figure out how to negotiate in group dynamics. It can help children learn how to compromise with others, recognise and respond to others feelings, how to share, show affection and resolve conflict. These social skills are important to help them form relationships.

Playing with other children helps them learn the art of communication. They come to recognise body language and facial expressions. They figure out how to start up conversations and how to express their thoughts and wants in a way that wont cause problems and put a stop to their group game.

Pretend play is especially important for children's communication and development. Role play gives children a chance to use words they have heard others use and can help improve their vocabulary.

Self directed play gives opportunities for children to use decision making skills. They can come across problems in a game and it can test their reasoning and judgment.

Yoga poses, games and activities should encourage their imagination and make believe play. This can be done in many ways like bringing in a theme to the yoga class each week, for example going on a journey to another country, meeting people that live there, seeing nature along the way and imagining you are a part of it, like a tree, having a pretend picnic, going to the beach and meeting some sea creatures, getting tired and then lie down and use the imagination to journey back to the class. Inventing stories involving the children and including poses to match the story, like animal poses and to encourage making noises like the animals is another great way to encourage their imagination.

Whether a make believe game or an arts and craft activity. Play provides children the freedom to explore new possibilities and to think up unique ideas as well as creative solutions to challenges they face. Active imagination will continue to serve children throughout their lives in an ever becoming complex world.

Children of this age group do have a short attention span and can tire quickly. Child development experts say that, on average, a 3 to 5 year old child should be able to stay focused on a task for two to five minutes times the year of their age, depending on the task. To help keep children's attention during a class an instructor could switch between fast and slow poses, games and activities, along with breathing and relaxation. Every time a change occurs the attention span should start form the beginning.

To help children keep focused, different creative tools could be used, for example whilst in a pose, counting or singing, or telling interesting animal facts and using sounds. Imagining being the pose could also help, for example being the animal of the pose, or being a seed when in child's pose and growing into a tree. Using props could also help, like a bean bag on the head for balancing poses.

This age group are so active that they can then become tired very quickly. This is normal for most children. Children can become tired usually for simple reasons, because they have been active, they need water or food, they haven't slept so well the previous night or they just need a little rest and recharge. After resting or refuelling children tend to recover and regain their energy just as quickly as they had become tired. Allowing time for water breaks, a quieter activity like a craft and imaginary relaxation could help in maintaining the children's energy and recovery.

Giving a variety of activities each week should help grab the children's attention and energy levels. Using ones voice when talking, like whispering or then being hyped up can help bring interest and energy to a class. Including lots of fun games and intertwining yoga poses into them should also help to keep that attention and energy during the class. Certain poses could be used to rest the body during the class, like Childs pose, or to bring energy, like a warrior pose. Every moment can be yoga and if an instructor is having fun then the children absolutely will too.

Children aged 3 to 5 years are finding their own feelings of awareness and independence and giving children time and space to explore this is honouring their intelligence. Children need to discover the world on their own and telling them to think in a certain way, or doing something better, or in a certain way is not optimising their learning experience. Providing a loving responsive and creative environment in a yoga class is allowing the children time to uncover their own truth.

It is more important for children to be able to be spontaneous and have fun whilst they are in a yoga pose and accuracy of the pose is not as important. If the children are safe in the pose and enjoying it, then there is no need to correct them. When a child feels that they are mastering a pose it can give them confidence and raise their self esteem. To correct a child in a pose can inadvertently be seen as criticism and can also take away their own chance of forming a relationship with the pose and working out in their own way what feels right for them.

Engaging children's minds by inviting them to become the pose can help encourage children to form their own relationship with the pose, for example, become a tree, grounding their routes into the ground and asking, can they stay there for hundreds or years.

To be open to children and allowing them to co create a yoga class together whilst at the same time keeping a basic structure of a class, can allow children time and space to flow in a way that can only happens in childrens play.

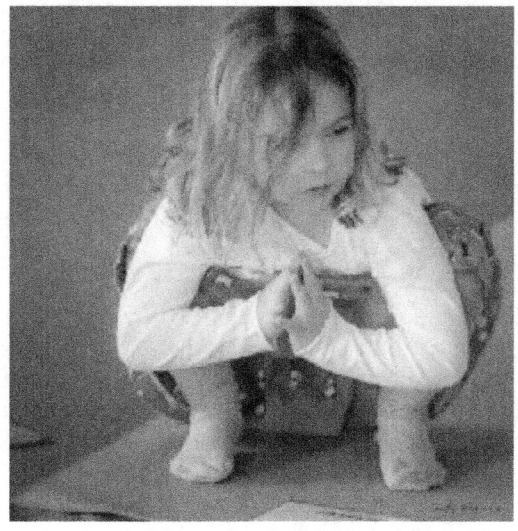

CHILDREN AGED 5-8

Children aged 5 to 8 years are rapidly growing. They are now free of development and physical limitations that much younger children experience and they are beginning to possess an increase in their own body awareness.

Their coordination has developed remarkably. They are active, agile and energetic and like to move around. Physical milestones for this age group are that they can now run, skip, balance well, climb, dance, jump, swing, and enjoy taking on any physical skill. An anything is possible attitude can be present in children of this age and they can believe that they can do anything and everything. Their motor skills, coordination and balance can allow them to do all sorts of yoga poses and sequences. They may begin to test their limits of their physical skills and it is important to help children to find their boundaries without pushing themselves too far and put themselves at risk of over stretching or over tiring themselves. A sign that a child may be pushing themselves to far is that their breathing becomes short and laboured.

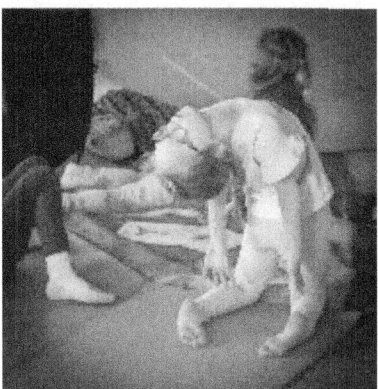

A good way of helping children find their limits and not going beyond them is to start where the children are at in their yoga practise and work up from there. Children of this age group may start noticing more differences of flexibility and strength in other children and a teacher can give easier and more challenging options for some poses, so that everyone feels successful. A yoga facilitator can emphasise that everyone is different and that this is an amazing thing, and, that people shine at different things. A teacher can also demonstrate their own limitations as an instructor so that children can feel comfortable with theirs.

Children of this age group may have at times, a lack of control over their energy and they can become more tired and irritable quickly. Poses and activities can be used to give periods of rest throughout the class to help.

Resting poses, such as Crocodile or Childs Pose could be used to help bring periods of rest, a craft activity or story is another way. Water breaks can help with resting and recharging energy too.

Children of this age group can be self confident and enjoy showing others their skills. There can be a desire to do well and be persistent in learning new skills. The class can now practise more challenging poses and games to meet this desire to learn new skills, whilst still keeping the class fun. However they can be self critical and have a need for approval. It is therefore important to take notice and praise them for their specific achievements.

They are more interested in other children now and can show friendliness and generosity. It is possible that this age group prefer rival games to team games. Yoga is non competitive and the spirit of this can be entwined in the class to help develop children's natural want of working with others. Partner or group poses and games that encourage non-competitiveness, cooperation and understanding of others can be used throughout a class to help develop this area.

Children are open now and ready to learn. Repetition in a class is now not required so much and this gradually gives way to an enjoyment of variation. Children of this age group will enjoy changes in activities and the introduction of new elements. Activities may need to be short and fast paced to match their energy and desire for challenges.

Children of this age group love challenges and one should allow themselves to be amazed by them.

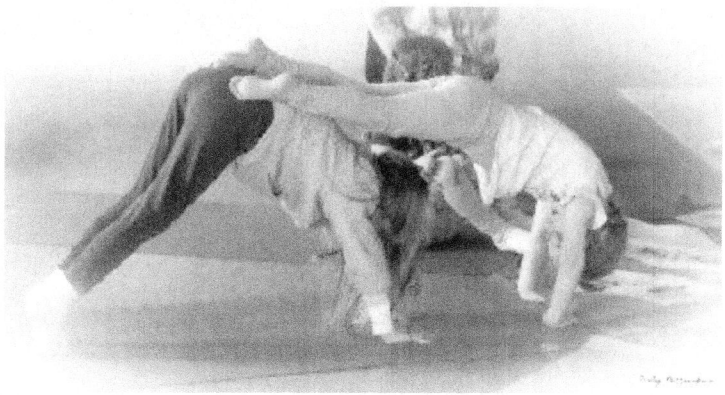

CHILDREN 8-11

Children aged 8 to 11 years physically are experiencing steady increases in their large muscle strength, balance and coordination and are now more coordinated. They now begin to experience growth spurts towards adolescence. They can be very active and have a lot of energy. Planning a yoga class for this age group may require more thought to make the class balanced to meet the children's energy and ability. Allowing time for a good warm up and then building the intensity of the poses gradually will encourage a safe practise for their physical bodies. It is important for this age groups growing and developing bodies to have a good diet and a good amount of exercise in their lives including a regular strengthening session.

As this age group have increased strength, balance and coordination, more emphasis can be on their technique now. More challenging yoga poses can be introduced to nourish their energy and ability. It is important for an instructor to provide any correction quietly. Children of this age group can be vulnerable to developing low body image. Helping children to connect with their body in yoga asanas and learning to enjoy and love them can help this age group to feel good about themselves. Talking about the physical and mental benefits of the poses is a way of helping children know that they are good for them and in what way. Their attention can be bought to specific muscles that are being stretched or strengthened in every pose. A good way to encourage awareness to their practise is to ask where in their bodies they feel the experience of the pose.

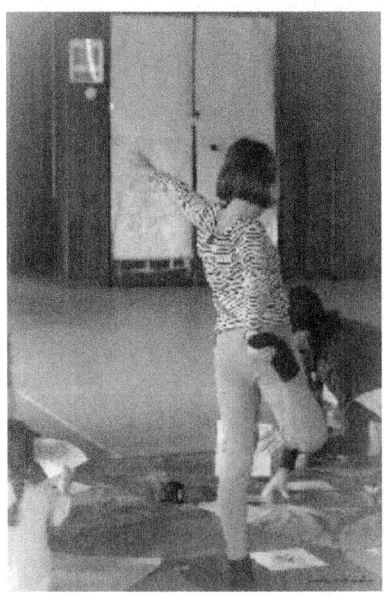

Giving positive feedback and looking for success can aid in developing their self confidence.

This age group may start to form stronger friendships and become more independent from parents and adults. They are more aware of being liked by others and may also seek approval from others. They may prefer to work in groups now, however they may find comparisons with other more difficult. This age group may have a more competitive nature especially towards gender groups. Promoting yoga's principles of non competitiveness in group work and activities is important to reinforce this and to encourage positive cooperative behaviour with each other.

Making this age group feel included in a group is a positive way of helping the children feel part of a group together. Allowing them to co-create a class together and letting them lead for a while is a good way of promoting their independence and ability to work together. An example way of doing this could be simply to put on some music the children like and take turns to lead a sequence of flowing poses. Discovering new ways of doing yoga together, like in partner sequence work, or creating a new yoga pose together is another way of promoting working together in a non competitive way.

Yoga for this age group needs to be interesting and relevant. Playing music that resonates with this age group to connect with them and as a group may bring opportunities to practise yoga and sequences based on their music. Introducing other elements like, arts, drama and yoga philosophy can offer more interesting areas to meet their increased concentration, intellect and creativity.

Group activities becomes important in a yoga session for this age group. Having a topic or theme for a class may help further in encouraging this. The topic can be anything, being strong or trusting the self and others, among many other topics. The whole session can be related to that topic, this can give a direction for the class and help to invite interest from the children. Yoga chanting, breathing exercises, warm up, asanas, games, activities and relaxation and meditation can all be around the chosen topic.

Movement, and therefore yoga, is essential for fast growing bodies of children aged 8-11 years. Yoga can also provide this age group with essential life tools such as self esteem and confidence, inner and outer strength , attention and concentration and heightened awareness of both oneself and others.

Children aged 8 to 11 years now have longer attention spans and are able to lie quietly for longer in relaxation and meditation.

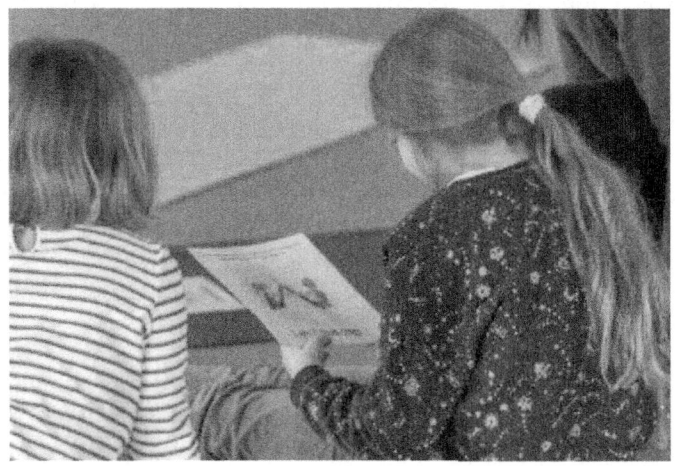

Studies have shown that teaching children mindfulness practices can build attentiveness, respect for others, self control and empathy, all while reducing stress, hyperactive behaviour and depression.

Giving tools to help fend of negative thinking and behaviours, build self confidence, focus, and treat others and themselves with respect and appreciation is a gift they will have for the rest of their lives.

CHILDREN AGED 11 +

While children aged 11 to teens are growing in all areas, in none is it more obvious than their social and emotional development. This age group want to be treated with respect and they deserve that. Trying to see their perspective may be able to help them in many ways through this major stage in their lives.

Puberty emerges around this age group, deeply effecting how individuals feel about themselves. They can develop a belief that others care intensely about their appearance and actions and can also believe that their personal experiences are unique. As a result of this children of this age can become highly self conscious, while at the same time feeling powerful and invincible. Listening and talking with the children about what they would like in their yoga class will help in making the class about them and their needs.

At this stage of development children can become aware of themselves as individuals and may work hard to be responsible and to accomplish more complex tasks. They can challenge the self confidence they have built over the preceding years and seek to find identity that they will take into adulthood. It can be a time for reflection of the sense of self. It can be a hard time for them where self esteem is concerned. A yoga class that includes breathing exercises, postures, relaxation and meditation techniques that encourages them to love and nurture the self and also to enjoy their physical bodies, can help continue to develop their confidence and self esteem in a positive way.

Adolescence may bring personality changes, that shows inconsistent behaviour, one minute they may be happy the next sad. It is time that they need patience, empathy and continued support in their lives. Breathing, relaxation and meditation for this age group can give them time for quiet in their busy lives and an opportunity to go within.

Relaxation skills for adolescents are essential. They can provide beneficial ways of dealing with stress. Research theorises that the mindful movement and breathing done in yoga activates the relaxation response. Therefore yoga can move an individual from the sympathetic nervous system, fight or flight state, into the parasympathetic nervous system, rest and digest state. It also increases neurotransmitters in the brain that helps the mind relax giving greater improvement in mood and anxiety. Yoga can be one of the most important and beneficial relaxation skills for adolescents.

Controlled breathing is one of the easiest ways to relax the nervous system and the most effective. Adolescents can learn to use deep breathing to help them relax and calm down when they may be feeling upset or stressed in their lives outside of the yoga class.

Research shows that mindfulness based exercises like yoga and meditation can help decrease anxiety, depression and stress. In turn this improves mental health and quality of life.

Friendships become vital for this age group and group identity starts to play a role in their lives. A competitive spark may continue to ignite and they may wish to dedicate more time and energy to particular hobbies and sports. Partner and group work that creates a non competitive environment is an important part of a yoga class for this age group. Allowing time for the students to work together and to be creative to add their own elements can bring feelings of accomplishment and empowerment.

This age group may become more interested in meditation, Sanskrit, the history and philosophy of yoga and therefore it can be a good time to incorporate this into a class. Finishing the sessions with inspiring quotes, poems or a question that they can carry with them into their lives and think about until the next session can aid in creating positive thinking. Even opening topics up for discussion if they want it and creating a safe environment for them to express themselves openly and be accepted for who they are.

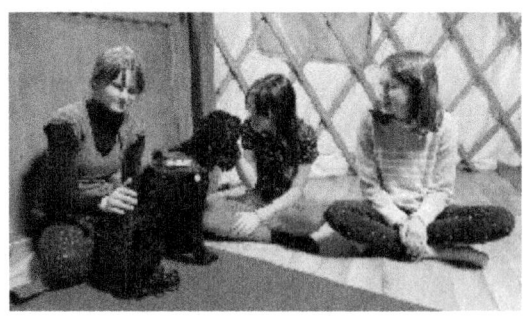

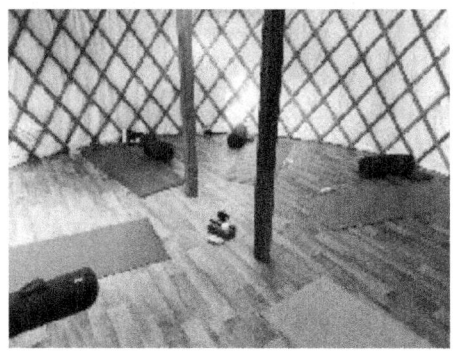

CHILDREN AND ADDITIONAL NEEDS

It is vital that the Yoga teacher is made aware of any child attending the class that has Special Educational needs such as a learning disability, speech and language impairment, autism or ADHD. The teacher can then ensure that their needs are met using strategies which successfully include students with special educational needs into the Yoga class. Here are some suggestions:

Begin and end the yoga class the same way every time.
Let the children know the plan for the lesson in advance and stick to it.
Offer a choice to the children, would they prefer choice 1 or choice 2.
Give a timely warning before you change an activity.
If children are asked to close their eyes, for example in relaxation or meditation, let them know how long for and that you will let them know when to open them again.
Develop a rapport with the children.
Offer alternative poses if needed and teach these visually and verbally.

Yoga has so many physical benefits for children particularly in promoting movement, increasing flexibility and easing aches, pains and joint stiffness. The practise can help relieve stress and equip children with the ability to better cope with their emotions. Children can learn how to use breathing and poses to calm down and it is these tools for self regulation and coping strategies that are especially useful for special education needs children and their carers. Practising yoga brings a feeling of accomplishment and achievement. As a consequence children feel more confident and in control of their bodies and emotions.

There are specific Yoga Teacher training courses available that will leave a yoga teacher well equipped to effectively share yoga with children with special and additional needs in a variety of settings.

Here we can take a deeper look at two conditions that may require additional support and care for a child in a yoga class.

Down Syndrome is a condition a person is born with, with an extra chromosome. Chromosomes contain hundreds, even thousands of genes. Genes carry information that develop our traits. With Down syndrome the extra chromosome causes delays in a way a child develops mentally and physically.

The physical features and medical problems associated with Down syndrome can vary widely from child to child. Some children with Down syndrome need a lot of medical attention, others lead healthy lives. The health problems with Down syndrome can be treated and many resources are available to help children and their families who are living with the condition.

Low muscle tone is a characteristic of children with Down syndrome, this can and does improve over time. Low muscle tone may also contribute to problems with feeding and constipation. Children with Down syndrome typically reach milestones like sitting up, crawling and walking later than some other children. Children with Down syndrome tend to grow at a slower rate and can be smaller than their peers.

Down syndrome affects children's ability to learn in different ways, but most have mild to moderate intellectual impairment. Children with Down syndrome can and do learn and are capable of developing skills throughout their lives. They simply reach goals at a different pace. Which is why it is important not to compare a child with Down syndrome against typically developing children. Children with Down syndrome have a wide range of abilities.

Studies have shown that yoga is beneficial with Down syndrome because it helps them improve muscle tone and flexibility while promoting a sense of inner peace. Yoga poses may also help internal organs and rejuvenate the endocrine glands. Simple breathing exercises help calm and restore the nervous system. For children with Down syndrome yoga helps bring body awareness and increases concentration and memory skills.

Yoga poses can be modified to meet any individual needs. Chanting, mantra repetition, mediation and relaxing to music are all ways to include additional holistic therapy into a yoga practise. The practises can maintain and restore mental, physical, emotional and spiritual health while encouraging creativity and self expression.

Breathing exercises are especially beneficial for children with congenital heart defects, common with Down syndrome. In addition they help ease pulmonary hypertension, relieve nasal congestion and build the immune system.

Yoga standing poses such as Mountain Pose, Tree Pose, Warrior Poses and Triangle pose can help to correct flat feet, weak angles and unstable knee caps as well as improve muscle strength through the body.

Thyroid dysfunction is also often a concern for children with Down syndrome. Yoga poses such as the bridge pose and shoulder stand can stimulate the thyroid gland. Twisting Poses can bring relief from digestive and constipation problems.

Yoga teaches relaxation skills through breathing techniques, meditation and poses. The relaxing pose of the Corpse can help to heal the body while inducing the relaxation response.

Sensory Integration Disorder is a condition in which the brain has trouble receiving and responding to information that comes into it through the senses. Some people with Sensory Integration Disorder are oversensitive to things in their environment. Common sounds may be painful or overwhelming. The light touch of a shirt may chafe the skin. Others with Sensory Integration Disorder may be uncoordinated, bump into things, be unable to tell where their limbs are in a space and find it hard to engage in conversation or play. Sensory Integration Disorder is usually identified in children but adults can also be affected.

Sensory Integration Disorder may effect one sense like hearing, touch or taste, or it may effect multiple senses. Children can be under or over responsive to the things they have difficulty with.

Like many illnesses, the symptoms of Sensory Integration Disorder exist on a spectrum. In some children for example, the sound of a leaf blower outside may cause them to vomit or dive under the table. They may scream when touched. They may recoil from the textures of certain foods. But others seem unresponsive to anything around them. They may fail to respond to extreme heat or cold or even pain. Many children with Sensory Integration Disorder don't handle change well. They may frequently throw tantrums or have meltdowns.

Therapists consider a diagnosis of Sensory Integration Disorder when the symptoms become severe enough to affect normal functioning and disrupt everyday life. Treatment for Sensory Integration Disorder is called Sensory Integration. The goal of Sensory Integration is to challenge a child in a fun, playful way so that he or she can learn to respond appropriately and function more easily.

Due to their heightened sensitivity to sensations or as a result of their motor based difficulties in individuals with Sensory Integration Disorder, they are more often than not in a constant state of alert. Yoga can help to bring them back into their bodies and learn to breathe, regulating their arousal levels and helping their central nervous system to relax. Through practising yoga, the asanas have so many wonderful benefits which help support the movement, body awareness, and touch sensory systems that can support an individual get back into their body and feed into their functional skills.

THE CLASSES

PLANNING THE CLASS

The basic structure of a children's yoga class should have elements of breathing exercises, postures, games and relaxation and these should be adhered to as much as possible. Other elements that can be included are music, storytelling, learning activities, role play and make believe, drawing and painting, eye exercises, singing and rhyming, visualisation, meditative awareness, yoga principles and yoga philosophy. A children's yoga class is normally around 45 to 50 minutes in duration with 10-15 minutes time for discussion or craft activities at the end. Breathing exercises are included in the first section, asana and games in the second and relaxation in the last.

Having a plan for the class ahead creates a secure environment for the child and also gives a teacher confidence for the session. Without a basic structure for the class, it can bring unfamiliar circumstances to a child and can potentially create stress for them.

A child will experience so much change in their lives, like trying new foods, changes in their education, and many more things, these changes often are not in their control. A class giving a familiar structure allows children to feel safe. It can also help them to develop mastery of their yogic skills when participating in a structured class. As this sense is strengthened it can help then to tackle larger changes in their own world.

It is still important to be spontaneous and creative in a class, there are times when a teacher will need to adapt, for example, a game is starting and the energy of the children have ideas for a different game. It is vital that the leader is open to the children's ideas, welcomes them, and adapts to meet their energy and direction. This openness and adaption shows the children that they are valued and that they are an important part of making the class a successful and an enjoyable one for all.

When planning each session for a children's yoga class an instructor needs to assess much information to ensure the class meets the needs and abilities of the children.

Having a theme when planning a class can help bring direction and creativity to developing an engaging class. Theme topics are plentiful, from nature, animals, the seasons, countries, cultures, religious festivals, emotional concepts such as mindfulness, yoga philosophy, national days, current events and happenings in the world that are meaningful are just some suggestions. The theme for a class could also compliment the relationship between yoga and learning subjects like maths, geography, history, science and physical education.

Having a theme for the whole term can also work well, an example of this could be, countries and cultures from around the world. Each week a country could be chosen and the class based around it. An example would be China, poses such as dragon pose or the various animals of the Chinese calendar could be included, a game that Chinese children play could be created, using colours of materials that represent China could be placed in the props basket, a Chinese folk tale could be told, music from China could be played, and a craft activity such as making Chinese lanterns. Connecting the children with children from other cultures brings natural qualities of interest, openness, understanding and acceptance of others.

Nature and animals are a beautiful topic to bring into a yoga class and it can encourage children to form or deepen their own relationship with the amazing world around them.

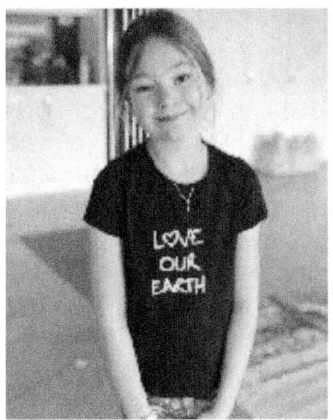

Children generally love animals and nature so it makes sense to introduce children to this ancient wisdom through something they love, making their learning relevant and meaningful. Just like the Yogis who invented yoga poses, children enjoy mimicking their surroundings through movement. Practising animal and nature yoga poses for children is an easy way for them to discover the physical postures of yoga.

Having themes that follow the energy of the seasons is also another great theme, this can help children deepen their relationship with nature whilst experiencing learning about the benefits of that when we live by the seasons we can receive natures healing balance, naturally and with ease, because each season has its own inherent balancing intelligence.

Stories are a really important area for children's language development and imagination. Having a story book, an idea of a story to tell, or some ideas of making up a story and acting it out with the children would be a creative way of bringing stories to the class.

We need inspiration to plan a class, which can sometimes feel challenging with so many choices, where do we start. You can find 52 planned children's yoga classes in this book to help or inspire you.

Here are some guidelines to help you in your planning.

Decide on a theme, to help you come up with one, consider what is going on around you, the time of year, seasonal festivities, special events such as the Olympic Games, special global days such as Earth Day, religious festivals such as Ramadan of Diwali all of these can help inspire you. Animal themed classes can be a favourite theme for children and there are so many individual themes on this such as, animals from certain countries, an African safari for example, or animals that are pets, animals that migrate or bring your favourite animal toy to class. Nature offers such a wide choice of enriching ideas, from the seasons, teaching of the laws of nature such as positive thinking attracts positivity, the many lessons that nature offers such as being able to let go when change is needed to grow like the fall of autumn leaves. Educational topics is another huge area to offer inspiration for classes, such as Countries of the World, Great Artists, Music from around the World, Historic events such as VE Day, Science experiments such as the concept of gravity, enriching stories that enhance the English language and mathematical shapes are just some examples. Emotional concepts such as mindfulness, coping with feelings of worry and anxiety, self esteem are some examples of the many important life skills that can be learnt in the yoga class. Yoga philosophy itself opens another door to the extensive range of inspiring themes for children's yoga classes, such as teaching from the mythology of the asanas or how to help calm the mind from busy thoughts through breathing and meditation exercises.

When you have decided on a theme, brainstorm what you already know about the theme and research any further information you need. Connect the theme with breathing exercises, games, postures, guided relaxation, stories and craft activities. Consider the energy curve to the class having a natural beginning, peak and end. Encapsulate your theme in a few key statements at the beginning and collect supportive words and phrases to continue linking the theme. Gather any inspiration readings or stories.

Finally, believe in yourself and trust your instincts.

ELEMENTS OF A CLASS

BEAUITFUL BEGININGS

The elements of a well-balanced children's yoga class can be split into three segments of 15 minutes each, to include, first segment of chanting, breathing exercises and breathing games. Second segment of warm up, yoga poses and games. Third segment of relaxation, meditative awareness and conclusion.

Chanting at the start of a class can help children relax and focus their attention for the session ahead. Chanting is sound and sound is a vibration of energy so by practicing chanting one can affect their energy field.

A mantra may be used in chanting, this can be any words in any language, or, words used from ancient Sanskrit. Sanskrit, the ancient Indian language which has also been found in ancient manuscripts from the Hindu, Buddhist and Jainism religions.

Mantra translates to, troubled mind free from, and it is a tool used to free one's mind. Repeating the word, Om, is a hugely beneficial mantra to begin using. Om, is believed to be the sacred sound of the universe and this belief stems from the Hindu religion, where it is believed Brahma's thoughts started a vibration that turned into, Om, and this is what lead to the creation of the world.

By harmonising our personal vibration with the vibration of the universal it can help one to connect with the self. This mantra can help calm the mind and the central nervous system. It also signifies unity and when used in a class it can help to bring a group together. Starting with chanting in a children's yoga class, can bring positive and happy feelings to the children and aid in their concentration.

It is believed that Sanskrit mantras work deeper to create lasting effects and healing and there are many ancient mantras that bring different effects.

The larynx, located in the throat, plays a major role in creating the sound of the voice. Two muscles, or the vocal chords, are stretched across the larynx and they are like rubber bands. When a person speaks, air rushes from the lungs and makes vocal chords vibrate which in turn produces the sound of the voice. The pitch of the sound produced is controlled by how tightly the vocal chord muscles contract as the air from the lungs hit them.

it is essential that the breath is relaxed and easy when practising chanting or singing. Having good alignment will help in ensuring no unnecessary pressure on the voice. Sitting or standing up straight with shoulders down and lengthening the neck will optimise the sound of the voice. Ensuring the abdomen and abdominal organs are relaxed will allow the lungs to fully expand. Chanting relies on the firm and steady out breath and allowing the lungs to fully expand will help in promoting this.

Creating an awareness of being gentle, soft and open in the throat, larynx and neck before and during chanting will help in not straining or restricting the voice. Yawning can help to open the throat and can give a child the opportunity to experience how the throat feels when it is open and relaxed. An open throat is intended to promote a type of relaxation in the throat and helps one to avoid constriction and tension whilst singing or chanting. An open throat is also believed to produce a sound quality that is round, open, free from tensions, pure rich, vibrant and warm in tone.

To explain opening the throat, children can be asked to sit down crossed legged with a straight back, shoulders down and neck straight. Ask the children to take a deep breath and then yawn. This action will open the throat. Children can be asked to bring their awareness to the feeling of their throat being open and that this openness will help them produce a good sound whilst singing or chanting.

Bending the neck forward constricts the throat and children can experiment with the sounds from their voice whilst they are doing this. It is important to not ask children to bend their heads backwards to ensure no risk of straining or injury to the throat or neck area.

It can also be explained that a good sound level whist chanting is, in a way that they can hear their own voice and others around them.

The voice is believed to be connected with the self, and this can be experienced when a person is feeling certain emotions, like fear or excitement, the quality of the voice changes. Just as emotions effect the quality of the voice, chanting can help promote a healthy voice.

INTRODUCE THE THEME OF THE CLASS

At the beginning of the class and after chanting, a welcoming and introduction of the theme of the class can be given. This can be a few sentences to explain what the class theme is about. Asking the children a question that is relevant to the topic is a way to help engage the children in it, this can also be an area of learning from each other and an insight into each child's knowledge on the theme.

Try to not overload all of the information about the theme in the introduction, rather give a brief explanation and then interweave information throughout the class within the segments. To do this make each segment relevant to the theme, if the theme is related to animals for example make the breathing exercise animal related and give some further information about that animal, do the same for the games, postures and relaxation, revisiting the theme and giving enriching and connecting pieces of information as the class develops.

BREATHING EXERCISES

It is wonderfully empowering for children to become aware of their own breathe and how to use it. When big emotions come, children can learn how to move themselves out of these reactive and encompassing states and back to a more relaxed feeling of rest.

To help children become aware of their breath, the practise of breathing exercises is needed. To practise such exercises when children are in a relaxed state, can help them harness their skills for moments outside of yoga when they may need it.

Slowing down and focusing on breathing is an immediate way to become aware of the breath. In a yoga class to practise breathing exercises, children can sit in a circle together to begin with and guidance can be given to help them get to know their breath by leading some breathing exercises.

Visualising is a useful tool to help children learn and practise breathing exercises, for example, balloon visualisation, sitting down or lying down, placing hands on the belly so that the belly can be felt moving with the breath. When breathing in, inflate the belly like a balloon and make it big. When breathing out, deflate the balloon pressing the abdomen to the back and squeezing all of the air out.

Using props is another useful tool to help children learn about their breath, using a feather or other item held in front of their nose and mouth and breathing in and out and seeing what happens to the feather.

Partner or group breathing exercises can also be done, an example of this is putting each others head or hand on another child's belly. When inhaling the head or hand is lifted and when exhaling the hand or head lowers.

Deep breathing also helps get rid of carbon dioxide, a waste product, and bring a better flow of oxygen to the body. Deep breathing can stimulate internal organs including the heart, bring fresh blood flow to the body carrying oxygen and nutrients to every cell as well as removing waste. It also calms the mind, reduces stress and provides a way of experiencing a greater holistic experience.

In yoga, breathing is primarily through the nose and also trying to use the abdomen as much as possible. Abdominal breathing is the natural breath. As individuals grow up, many start to breathe primarily with the chest and forget how to breathe with the abdomen.

Lungs have a triangular type shape with the wider part at the bottom. When breathing with the chest only the breath is shallow. There is more space at the bottom of the lungs and more air sacs there to receive oxygen from the air and bring it into the blood stream. Abdominal breathing massages inner organs and the heart with movement of the diaphragm and is a deeper more efficient breathing.

Deep breathing also affects the nervous system. When the nervous system is operating with everything as normal, the breath naturally uses the abdomen to breathe. When stress or anxiety occurs, the breath automatically switches to chest breathing. Breathing using the abdomen switches on the relaxed nervous system and helps bring feelings of calm and brings the body back to harmonious function.

Teaching older children how to breathe using the abdomen and the effects it can have physically and emotionally on the body is an important part of a class.

Children should not be asked or taught to hold their breath whilst performing breathing exercises. Children's bodies are developing and growing and to restrain and hold the breath requires physical strength and energy.

CHILDREN'S BREATHING EXERCISES WITH INSTRUCTIONS

Airball Game
Straw and cotton ball/paper/feather. Lie on tummy in circle facing in. Pass the ball around the circle blowing through straw.

Air Walk
Lie on back. Inhale lift right leg and left arm, exhale and lower. Inhale, lift left leg and right arm, exhale and lower. Keep going, inhale in time with lift and exhale as you lower. Keep legs and arms straight.

All Good Things
Think of things that make you feel good such as fun, kindness, focus and confidence. As you speak and repeat the movements three times, feel those good things.
All good things ...
Rain down on me - raise your arms scoop them in, press them down in front of you.
Grow up through me - scoop your hand in and up together to your heart
Surround me - push your hands forward and around your body as if you are doing breast stroke.

Alternate Nostril Breath

Revitalising, help to concentrate and can bring clarity and equanimity to both sides of brain. This is a great exercise to practise pre an exam or similar situation. Breath that calms the mind. Left nostril represents calm, cooling and feminine. Right side represents force and masculine. Said to balance both hemispheres of brain. Exhale the breath through both nostrils. Use the right hand, thumb and ring finger, close right nostril using right thumb, inhale left, exhale right nostril whilst closing left nostril with ring finger. Inhale right nostril, close right nostril with right thumb, release ring finger to exhale left nostril. Repeat cycle.

Back Breathing

Encourages awareness of breath in back. Sit against wall, bring awareness to the movement in the back whilst breathing in and out. This exercise can be practised in partner work with one child sitting on the heels, whilst the partner sits behind with hands on partners back feeling how the breath moves the back.

Back to Back

Working with a partner, sit on the floor cross legged and back to back. Place the hands on the knees and close the eyes. Feel the support of each other. Notice if you can feel your partner breathing. (pause) Try not to force the breath, let it be natural. (pause). See if you can match your partners breath. (pause). We have so much to be grateful for, we can be grateful for our breath.

Balloon Breath is a simple breathing exercise in yoga that can help children feel relaxed and calm. Balloon breath can also help children to become more aware of the movement of their breath, experiencing the depth and breadth of it and how it can make them feel. Practising breathing deeply can help children experience the benefits of bringing feelings of calmness and or creating more blood flow around their body for more energy and that they can then use the practise when they may need it in their lives.

To practise Balloon Breath, children can be asked to sit comfortably in a cross legged position with their back straight. To close their eyes and imagine a soft round balloon in their tummy. Children can be asked to describe what colour their balloon is to help them really connect with the exercise. To place their hands on their tummy and imagine holding the balloon. To breath in through the nose and imagine the balloon filling up. Then breathing out slowly through the nose and feel the balloon going down and the tummy flattening. This exercise can be repeated five or six times and the children can be asked how it felt. Balloon Breath, can also help children become aware of their abdominal breathing.

Bear Breath
In winter bars hibernate in caves, sleeping peacefully, children can discover their own inner peace with this breathing exercise. To practise children can be instructed to sit up tall, close the eyes and go inside. Breathe in through the nose, inhaling for a count of five. Then breathing out for a count of five. Repeat this exercise for five to seven rounds. Asking the children to open their eyes and notice how they feel.

Bee Breath
Sit cross legged and comfy. Part teeth keep mouth closed, inhale, close both ears with index finger as breathe out through nose make a humming sound in throat. Keep jaw relaxed. Repeat 5 times. Bees hum their days away visiting flowers and making honey. Children can be asked as they hum to think of what makes them happy.

Bird Breath
Calming and grounding. Sit or stand. Breathe in through nose as bring arms out to side and up over head, breathe out through nose as lower arms like bird wings. Repeat several times. Take flight if you so wish.

Breathing Staircase
Group breathing exercise. One child lies on back, eyes closed, knees bent, feet flat on floor. Next child lies at right angles head on tummy, next child same and so on. First child beings a regular pattern of breathing, second child listens and feels breathing and matches breath and so on until whole staircase is breathing in unison.

Bunny Breath
Sit on heels, back straight shoulders wide. Three times sniffs in then exhale through nose. Bunnies are alert, this exercise can bring alertness.

Cocoon Breath
Pretend to be a caterpillar snug in chrysalis or cocoon. Take deep long breaths in and out, transform into butterfly or moth, fly around if so wish.

Candle Breath
Sitting in a comfortable position with spine tall. Interlock hands with index fingers up. Imagine holding a candle in the index fingers, inhale the exhale through the mouth gently blowing out the flame on the candle, repeat 2 or 3 times. Then repeat the exercise breathing through the nose.

Complete Breath
Sit up tall with one hand resting just below the belly button, the other hand on chest. Relax face, shoulders and abdomen. Inhale slowly through nose, filling belly first, then ribs, then chest, pause. Exhale slowly out of nose from

upper chest first, then rib cage, then belly. Repeat several times. Complete breath gives an internal workout.

Cooling Breath
Sitting with the spine tall, shoulders relaxed. Roll the tongue inwards to make a tube shape. If you find this difficult bring the teeth close together. Breathe in through the mouth, in through the tongue or teeth, feel the cool air go through the tongue and down into the body. Relax the tongue, close the mouth and exhale slowly through the nose. Continue for a few breaths.

Cotton Ball / Feather
Sit in a circle, place cotton ball on hand, hold under nose, inhale, exhale through nose watch what happens to ball. Experiment with the breath, inhale and exhale through the mouth what can the chid see happening to the ball.

Count to Five Breath
Sitting in a comfortable position, relaxing tension Open one hand, take deep breath in through nose, exhale, fold down thumb, count 1, breathe in then exhale fold down 1 finger count 2, continue to 5.

Didgeridoo Breath
Inhale, exhale like playing the didgeridoo.

Different Ways of Breathing
Breathe through nose, mouth, hands. Hands feel cold blow fingers, hands feel hot haa. Yawn, sigh. Pant like a dog, hoot like an owl, whistle like a bird.

Dragons Breath
Fists under chin, inhale, exhale sharply with tongue out as move arms down like breathing fire.

Easy Breath
Sit in a comfortable position eyes closed. Imagine the belly is the ocean and the breath the waves. As the waves roll in, breathe in, as the waves roll out, breath out. Allow the breath to be natural and easy, flowing effortlessly. Just watch it happen like the ocean at the beach enjoy becoming more and more relaxed and peaceful. When one breathes into the belly instead of the chest, a message is sent to the body to relax.

Elephant Breath
Elephants can shower themselves with their own trunks. Instruct the children to choose something to shower themselves with, sparkles, love, laughter, strength. Stand with feet wide apart. Link hands and dangle arms

in front of body like an elephant trunk. Inhale through nose as raise arms high above the head and lean back. Exhale through the mouth as arms swing down through the legs. Repeat for three rounds. On the next round stay up, arch back and shower yourself.

Full Breath
Sit or stand with spine erect, hands on rib cage. Inhale deeply and feel ribs move up and out. Exhale slowly and feel ribs move down and in. Repeat x 4.

Green Breath
Sit outside surrounded by nature or inside by a window. Notice the green trees, grass and flowers. Close eyes, slowly breathe in oxygen. Imagine being filled with green energy that feels healthy and alive. Slowly exhale. Imagine the carbon dioxide being breathed out filling the plants with well being. Repeat several time. Children can be directed to imagine that they are breathing friends with the plants.

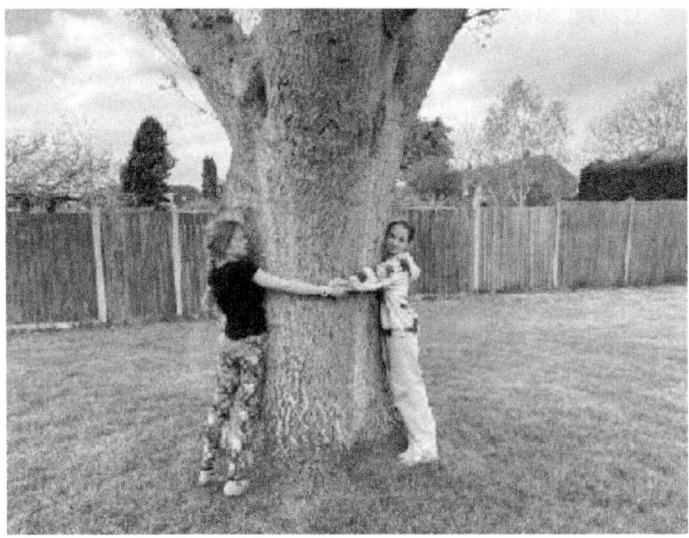

Heart Mudra
Make a heart shape with the hands, place hands by the heart, inhale exhale. Inhale love, exhale love to friends, inhale then exhale to family, then animals, plants, yogis and finally the world.

Hot Air Balloon
A good wake up breathing exercise. Sit on the heels, inflate tummy and lungs by taking little sips of air whilst raising the arms up, little by little, until over head. Once filled deflate, relax body to ground. Relax in a gentle heap.

Inhale Good Thoughts
Children can be instructed that they can breathe in good thoughts and then try it, Inhale something good like, I like myself, I am capable, I can do it. Repeat.

Joy Breath
Stand with your feet apart, knees slightly bent keeping arms straight. Inhaling raise both arms up above head, exhale lower arms to chest level, inhaling open arms to the side, exhaling bring arms back to the middle, inhaling bring arms up over head, exhaling strongly and sharply with a HAAAH sound. Bend knees and swing arms down and behind body. Then swing them up as inhale to begin again. Repeat three to five times. Then close the eyes and notice how feel, happier, lighter, invigorated?

Lion Breath, could be included as a breathing exercise for a theme of, Wild Animals, in children's yoga. It can relieve tension and stress. Lions breath stretches the entire face including the jaw and tongue. Lions breath can remind us not to take yoga too seriously. It is a good exercise to practise first thing in the morning to warm up and increase energy.

Lions breath can be practised from kneeling whilst sitting on the heels. Placing the hands on the knees, straightening the arms and extending the fingers. Inhaling through the nose, exhaling strongly through the mouth making a, ha, sound. Like a roar of a lion. As opening the mouth wide, stick out the tongue as far as possible towards the chin. Inhale and return to a neutral face. This exercise can be repeated.

Ocean Breath
Sit up tall. Relax face, shoulders and belly. Close eyes. Touch the top of the tongue to the roof of the mouth. Inhale through the nose for 3-4 counts. Exhale out of opened mouth for 4-8 counts and say haah. Imagine the sound of the ocean. Repeat 3-5 times. Ocean breath is a soothing breath.

Pinwheel Breath
Practise blowing pinwheel with variations. Notice how pinwheel reacts.

Peace Breath
Close eyes, relax face muscles. Inhale, on exhale whisper word, peace. Do this 3-6 times. As you say the word feel peace inside you. Exhale send peace to - animals, trees, plants, family, friends, world.

Prop on Tummy
Lie on back, notice which parts of body move whilst breathing. Place prop on tummy, watch. Explain that fully breathing expands the tummy and that breathing this way can then move the prop more.

Rainbow Breath
Sit cross legged with hands on knees. Inhale, arch back and look up. Exhale round back and look down. Repeat 7 times, breathing each shade of the rainbow…. Red, orange, yellow, green, blue, indigo, violet. Rainbow breathe cleans and brightens the whole body.

Roller Coaster Breath
Raise hand to face, start at the thumb, inhale use finger or other hand to move up thumb, exhale continue finger over thumb and down, inhale next finger and repeat until at end of hand.

Side Breathing in yoga the exercise gives the experience and teaching of expanding the rib cage and back to allow for a full intake of air into the lungs. To practise side breathing lie on the right side and place the left hand on the lower ribs area. Breathe in slowly and deeply and feel the rib cage spreading apart and the hand rising with the breath. Breathe out slowly and repeat several times. Turn onto the other side and repeat the exercise.

Side breathing can sometimes be referred to as lateral breathing, which emphasise the lateral expansion of the rib cage. The ribs move outward and upward. This breathing exercise can mobilise the rib cage. All joints within the rib cage are designed to move, so deep thoracic breathing gets the rib cage to its fullest potential, a rib cage this is stiff can impede breathing.

Sitting Back to Back
With a partner sit back to back, link arms, take deep breaths in through the nose and out of the mouth. Be mindful of partners breath.

Snake Breath
When they are coiled and resting, snakes look around calmly, and when they move, they are slow and smooth. Sit up tall. Take a deep breath in, filling up the whole body. Pause and breathe out slowly and smoothly, making a hissing sound for as long as can. Repeat for three to five rounds, feeling the self slow down and become calmer each time.

Sounding Breath
Sit up tall. Relax the face. Lengthen the back of neck. Open mouth. Breath in and out making a haah whispering sound. Now close the mouth and continue to breathe slowly in and out of the nose making that same haah

sound. Cover the ears, close the eyes and listen. Sounding breath is calming. Yogis use it to help them stay focused.

Sun Breath
Inhale, lift arms out and up, exhale hands to heart. Repeat saying thank you to the sun for a new day.

Train
Have a train ride to ….. Sit one behind the other cross legged, make fists with the hands hands and tuck arms into sides of body. Inhale through the nose and punch one arm out in front, exhale punch other out and first arm back in. Keep on breathing forcefully in and out as continue to switch arms. Listen to the sound of the breath. Breathe in and out as the train arrives at station.

Triangle Breath
Inhale draw one side of triangle using finger in front of you, exhale other side, inhale line at bottom. Continue.

Twist and Breath
Helps understand breath and movement coordination. This is a good transition exercise into a warm up activity. Lie back knees bent feet flat on the floor, arms out to the sides palms facing up. Breath in then out through the nose whilst dropping knees to right turn head to left. Inhale bring knees to chest, exhale drop knees to left and turn head to right. Repeat x 5

Warrior Breath
Standing feet hip distance apart knees soft arms by side. Repeat to self, "I am strong". Repeat "I am ready", whilst inhaling tuck elbows in with fists facing up. Repeat "I punch sharply" whilst exhaling though the nose and punch forward turning the fist down. Repeat "I am fiery" whilst Inhaling bringing the arm back into the side of the body. Exhale and punch other fist and arm forward. Repeat for several rounds at a fast pace, then rest and feel the inner fire.

Woodchopper When there is tension, frustration, anxiety or anger in the body it needs to be released. The Woodchopper Pose, is an excellent tool for children to release tension in a controlled and safe manor. The, Woodchopper, helps reduce stress from the body and mind with movements of the arms in a swaying motion. The major muscles in the body are activated resulting in the flow of fresh blood in the body encouraging children to feel energetic and light. The pose benefits the arms and shoulders, lower and middle back, the biceps and triceps, chest, hips and knees.

The use of the mouth to breathe out the stale air whilst breathing in through the nose helps to release stress and tensions. When breathing out through the mouth, more air is expelled and encourages more air in on the inhalation. This brings more fresh and oxygenated air into the lungs which is believed to bring more energy to cells in the body.

As well as the release of tension and physical benefits of the Woodchopper Pose, it can also be used as a vehicle for creating positive self talk by replacing negativing feelings with positive. When breathing in, a positive thought can be taken in replacing the negative feeling which can be released on the out breath. This can be a first step in developing a growth mindset, taking in the positive and releasing the negative.

To practise Woodchopper Breath, clasp the hands together in front of the body. Take a long breath in while raising the hands above the head. Exhale vigorously with the mouth open making a, haaa sound while swinging the arms down between the legs as if chopping wood. Hang the head and completely let go of all the tension in the body. Repeat the exercise.

WARMING UP THE BODY & MIND

It is really important to warm up the body before practising Yoga asanas. Warming up the body with movements and gentle stretches increases the, cardio vascular system, raises the body temperature and increases blood flow to the muscles. Warming up before physical activity can help to reduce muscle soreness and lessen any potential risk of injury. It can also optimise the ability of the muscles to perform.

By warming up, the muscles become prepared for physical activity ahead, this is due to the increase in their elasticity, tension being reduced, and the willingness to exercise them is intensified. It is advisable to increase the level of activity gradually and to not do the fullest expression of each to begin with.

A warm up should be fun and engaging for the children, this will help clear their minds and prepare them. A fun warmup can also grab children's interest for the class ahead. The warm ups should be changed to ensure that children get a variety and that they don't do the warm up from repetitiveness or memory.

Warm up exercises, games and Sun Salutations are great ways to warm the body prior to the postures section of the class. Here are some suggestions for warm up activities and games for this section of the class.

WARM UP ACTIVITY AND GAME IDEAS

Bake a Cake
Sit on floor with crossed legs or in butterfly or wide leg sitting positions. Reach up for ingredients, put into bowl, stir. Ask each child what is in their cake.

Beach Volley Ball
Write warm up instructions on a ball or beach ball that connect with the oceans or beach such as, starfish jumps, crab walks, turtle crawls, dolphin jumps, jellyfish swimming, kelp forest swaying in the ocean, rock. Throw the ball to each other, wherever the catcher right thumb lands do that warm up activity.

Catch the Butterfly
In this game, children can enjoy being both quick and delicate like a butterfly. Form partners and find a leaf. Choose a thrower and a catcher. The thrower tosses the leaf in the air for the catcher who tries to catch it as though it

were a butterfly, gently with open palms. When the catcher is successful switch roles.

Chinese Dragon Dance
Dragon asleep -sit on floor rock head up and down side to side, wake up - jump up stretch arms up high and tilt head to side to side, bow - 3 times, explore - walk around and pretend you are looking for something, freestyle, test food, find and inspect food and then jump back repeat from different angles, eat food - pretend to eat food with paw, share luck - keep chomping then throw your food at friends to catch, lick - pretend to lick yourself by sliding head down each leg twice, bow - 3 times, sleep - sit on floor slowly rock head up and down side to side.

Circle of Friends
Stand shoulder to shoulder in a circle facing inwards. Make eye contact and appreciate your friends. One player stands in the middle, arms length away from the circle, feet together, arms crossed over chest, body straight and stiff. Friends stand with one leg back and one forward, elbows bent, hands up. Middle player leans over and is gently passed across and around the circle. Friends give support that is strong yet gently firm yet caring.

Don't wake the Dragon
One player becomes the sleeping dragon and the other players become villagers or knights. Place any small object representing the magic key, close to, but not touching the dragon. One at a time, villagers sneak up and try to retrieve the magic key without waking the dragon. Making any noise or touching the dragon will trigger her or him to wake and roar a fiery breath. Being successful at retrieving the object requires a lot of finesse. If a player wakes the dragon, her/his turn ends. When a player gets the magic key without disturbing the dragon, she/he becomes the dragon and a new round begins.

Earth Missions
Warm up with moving around the room, ask the children to suggest alternative ways to travel that doesn't pollute the planet, such as walking to the shops rather than use a car, skip, run, cycle, row a boat…. Move around the room demonstrating that mode of travelling.
Plant trees, working in pairs, one child to take Childs Pose as a seed of a tree, the partner tends to the tree, waters it and helps it to grow into a tree, (Tree Pose), ask the children what tree they have grown into. Swap over so that the other partner gets a turn to grow into a tree.
Pick up Rubbish, using marbles and a hula hoop, spill the marbles inside the hoop, the children can pick up the pretend rubbish using their toes and placing them in a cup.

Reduce, Reuse, Recycle mantra, repeat three times in the following poses Upward Facing Dog (reduce) into Downward Facing Dog (Reuse) into Plank (recycle).

Easter Egg Hunt
Hide eggs with warm up instructions attached, such as 10 bunny hops, 10 spring leaps, 10 windmill arms etc… Children take turns to go find an egg and bring back to group for children to perform.

Emotion Exploration
Draw or write various emotions on card, happy, angry, excited, disgusted, angry, sad, scared etc…. Invite the children to pick a card and then show everyone what emotion they have picked. Ask the children to take a moment to think about that emotion and if it were a movement how would that look. After a count of 3 each child demonstrates their move for that emotion. Pick one child each turn to show the group their move, ensure all children get a turn at this.

English Folk Dance
Play traditional music, beat x 16 counts, clap, swing arms, march, walk, skip, jump. Partner or group right hands in for right hand turn, repeat for left, spin move one person crosses arms other straight spin, change so other child crosses arms spin in other direction.

Fairy Ring Dance
Have two rows of children lined up facing each other. Take four skips towards each other and four skips back, repeat. Take four skips towards each other and all hold hands to make a circle. Take eight gallops to the right and then eight gallops to the left. Skip back four skips to return back to where started. Repeat as many times as the children like.

Feather Race
Divide into relay teams and give each player a straw and a feather. Designate a start and a finish line. Place your feather on the ground. On go, players blow through the straws to move their feather across the finish line. As soon as one player crosses the next team member follows until everyone has finished. After the game turn to friend and take turns brushing the feather on each others face. Notice how your body and breathing relax.

Firefly Dance
Ask the children to bring a head torch or small torch to class. Make the room as dark as possible. Light the torches and be fireflies dancing in the night sky.

Freeze Yoga

Play some fun music, children move or dance around, when the music is paused, the children freeze in a yoga pose. You can also theme this game such as nature poses or Christmas pose, or a theme of your choice.

Go Stop Back to Back
Appoint a leader. Spread out. Follow directions, go walk, go crawl, go skip, go roll etc…. When leader calls stop back to back, stand or sit back to back with another person. Play lively music.

Go With the Flow
Make an assault course for the children. Each child completes the course holding a glass of water trying not to spill or waste any water. Use the mats for lily pads, skipping rope to walk along and to balance, use a balance pose at a station, step over blocks etc…. Don't forget to ask the children to use the water for a drink for a plant so not to waste this precious life giving source.

Hula Hoop Challenge
Set up hula hoops to make a hopscotch assault course. The children can jump with 1 foot between two or on one foot on one.

Gratitude Activity
Split group in 2. 1 group stands in circle, close eyes. Second group listen to prompts given by teacher, then this group silently go around and touch each person in the circle gently on the shoulder, they can go to more than one person. Talk about how might feel if not get touched and how we might prevent anyones feelings getting hurt. Suggested prompts can be, a person that has smiled at you, works hard, has shown gratefulness, you are grateful for, made you laugh, doing their best, fun to be around, you admire.
Talk about how it felt to be a receiver / giver.

Hula Dance
Play music and dance the Hula. Begin with side steps to the right and then repeat in other direction. Then introduce hips. Then introduce arms rolling arms like waves of the ocean.

Human Knot
This warm up game takes practise in being kind, gentle, supportive and cooperative. Stand in a circle facing inwards. Reach out and take hold of two different peoples hands, left hand to left hand and right hand to right hand. Do not take hold of anyones hand that is next to you. Begin to untie the human knot together so that you are standing in a circle holding hands.

Icebergs

Using two sheets place them on the floor away from each other. Divide the children into two teams. The sheets can be anything from icebergs melting to grassland habitats shrinking. Play music have the children move around the room, when the music stops each team have 10 seconds to be on the sheet. Each turn the sheet is folded in half getting smaller and smaller until the children are unable to all be on the sheet. Children can lift each other off of the floor, it is advisable not to have any children go onto another shoulders or above this height.

Jazzy Jamming
Sit in a circle. Be a group of musicians about to create a piece of music using voices and hands to sing, hum, whistle, clap, knock etc…. Close eyes and listen carefully. Notice the sounds around and the silence. When ready, choose a theme to inspire the music, e.g rainforest, party, winter….
Appoint a leader to start the rhythm or melody, weave in sounds as the children feel moved. Allow the music to arise and die away naturally. Share a few moments of silence at the end, then open eyes and thank one another.

Jump the Mats
Have the mats in a circle. Using a small hand drum, beat different number of sounds on the drum, the children jump the number of mats beaten.
(Invented by Bella)

Love Train
Children make a line one behind the other. Play music, use any props such as scarfs for the children to hold. The leader of the line moves around the room leading the group moving freely, they may wish to walk, skip, run, dance, the rest of the children follow the leader. After a short time indicate the leader going to the back of the train of children and the next child becomes the leader. Continue until all children have a turn at leading the train.

Moon Salutations
Similar to sun but practise with a side bend in a crescent moon shape.

Musical Mats
Yoga card placed on each mat. Play music when music stops children find a mat and perform yoga pose displayed.

Musical Yoga Dots
Place Yoga cards under mat dots, play music, when music stops children find a dot, read the pose and practise it on the dot.

Nature Kids

Make a list of natural phenomena such as storms, clouds, trees, rainbows, waves, fire etc…. Spread out. Appoint a leader to call out the words in any order at any speed. Act out each of the words in the way you think is best.

Over and Under
Divide into relay team lines. On go the front of each line passes the ball or water balloon over their head to the next player who passes it under their legs to the next who passes around them to the next who starts the pattern again. When the ball or balloon reaches the last player she or he runs to the front of the line and passes it over their head. The first team to have the original players standing at the head of the line wins.

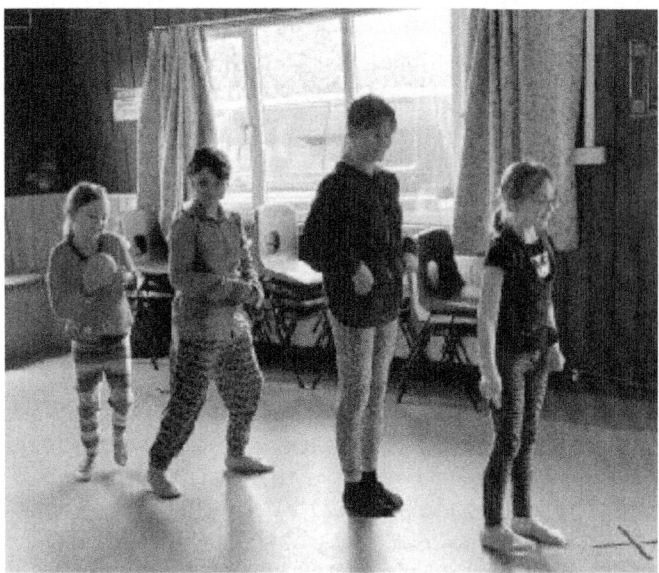

Partner Mash Up
Play music guide the children to move or dance around the room. When the music stops each child finds the closest partner. State the instruction picked and the children follow the instruction. Instruction ideas - Noodle soup, one child places their hands and arms around their partner whilst their partner spins around in their arms. Dog in a dog house, one child performs Downward Facing Dog pose, their partner lies on the tummy under the pose. Bird on a perch, one child kneels on the floor with one knee up, their partner sits on their knee. London Bridge, both children bring their palms together above their heads to make a bridge shape. Being creative with ideas of your own to add to the selection or theme.

Pass the Torch

Divide into relay teams. Mark a start and finish. Each team gets piece of felt as their torch. One at a time, players move quickly to the finish line and back with the torch on their heads. They then pass the torch to the head of the next player without using their hands. If the torch falls off it must be put back by the player or someone from his or her team without using any hands. Toes, feet and elbows may all be used. The first team to have the original player standing at the front of the line wins.

Pollinators Game
Half the children to be flowers or plants and take flower pose sitting on their mats, the other half of the children will be bees or pollinators. The children in flower pose can decorate themselves with pollen using bean bags, scarfs or any other suitable items. Play music whilst the pollinator children fly around the flowers and plants taking items (pollen), they can leave some items on other flowers, when they have collected enough pollen they return to their hive (yoga mat) to deliver it to the hive. Swap over so that the flowers can be pollinators too.

Rock Tree Bridge
First child becomes a rock, second child steps over the rock and makes a tree, third child steps over the rock, walks around the tree and makes a bridge. 4th child steps over the rock, walks around the tree and crawls under the bridge to then make a rock. Repeat the pattern of rock tree bridge.

Runaway Reindeers
Santa is tagger, chases reindeers. If caught go into star pose, to free the reindeer another child needs to go under legs. Quiet come to mat for sleeping reindeer pose (rock). Take turns to be Santa.

Spinning
Whirling Dervishes. Stand in Mountain Pose, take arms out to the sides, start slowly, spin faster and faster then slow down. Play music.

Trees & Wind Game
Half children take Tree Pose, half the children are the wind. Winds cant touch the trees, they can move around the trees to create wind to try to blow over the trees.

Trick or Treat
Get costumes on, shake and move body. Set up stations with yoga cards or warm up instructions, as a group visit the stations, read the card or instruction, is it trick or treat. Ideas to perform, hop scotch dots, bean bag throw, tight rope walk, warm up exercise or will there be a treat.

VE Day Swing Jive
Learn the basic steps to the swing jive and practise to music

Wheelbarrow Races
Make teams. Have items at one end of the room that match the theme of the class, such as healthy play food. Teams make a line behind each other. The first child moves onto their hands whilst the child behind them takes hold of the front of their shins or ankles making a wheelbarrow. The wheelbarrow needs to get to the end of the room to collect an item and return it to the team for the next two children to go. Play stops when every child has had a turn and all of the items are collected.

Yoga Assault Course
Set up mats as stations with Yoga Cards on each mat. Use bean bags, skipping ropes, egg & spoon for balance and mindfulness between stations.

Yoga Limbo
Use skipping rope or item for the limbo bar, play music, children do poses or movements under bar such as crawl, crab walks, frog walks, snake slides. Lower the bar each round.

Yoga Pretzels
Stand apart from each other, loose and relaxed. Choose a leader. Leader calls out the names of body parts. The players have to make shapes by letting only these body parts touch the floor. E.g one foot and one thumb, one knee and one elbow, two knees, tummy, shoulders and feet etc…. Be sure to take turns as leader. For more of a challenge play in pairs.

Yogi Says
Choose a leader and play just like Simon Says. Leader demonstrates different movements or yoga poses. Players follow along only when leader says, Yogi says. If leader does not say players that moved must perform a consequence chosen by the leader. Leader chooses a yoga pose or something fun like a donkey kick or frog jump. Then choose another leader. Take turns being the leader. Try giving directions for group formations like yogi says everyone make a flower or a star.

Yoga Tag
Tagger catches others by gently touching with a soft ball or toy, that person is then the tagger. If a child is in a yoga pose they are safe and cannot be tagged.

SUN SALUTATIONS

Sun Salutations, known as Surya Namaskar in Sanskrit, are designed to warm the body and spine to prepare for the yoga postures that follow. It is a graceful sequence of 12 postures that flow seamlessly into each other. Surya means sun and Namaskar means to bow too. Traditionally Sun Salutations are practised in the morning with the rising sun shining on and warming the spine. The sequence can vary somewhat between yoga schools.

For children, practising Sun Salutations can be fun and has many benefits, they can help to calm the mind and bring focus, energise the body and boost endurance, increase strength and flexibility and introduces linking breath to movement.

A fun element can be integrated into practising Sun Salutations and the order of the postures and transitions can be adapted to match the theme of the class and the children's level of ability. Practising to music can also invoke flowing of movement and synchronises the sequence with others.

Below is a basic Sun Salutation sequence for children that can be adapted, themed and developed as the children progress in their practise.

Begin in Mountain Pose, inhale stretch arms up towards the sky, reach tall.

Exhale take the arms out to the sides and dive forward into standing forward fold.

Place the palms on the floor and step back into plank position.

Inhale and gently drop the knees to the mat. Exhale tuck the elbows in towards the body and lower down to the mat in one straight line.

Inhale lifting the chest, shoulders and head into Baby Snake Pose. Exhale roll the chest and arms back to the mat.

Inhale place the palms on the mat next to the chest, push down on the palms, lift the hips up and back into Downward Facing Dog.

Exhale bend the knees look forward and either step or jump the feet to the hands coming into Standing Forward Fold.

Inhale the arms back up to the sky reach tall. Exhale the arms to the sides standing in Mountain Pose.

ASANAS / POSTURES

Asanas form the main part of the session. There is no specific order for the postures, however a good balance for an all over mind and body experience should be included.

For children, postures can really be bought to life, a child can fully immerse themselves into them, they can imagine they are a tree or a cat helping to further develop their imaginative and creative skills.

Practising Yoga postures for children can help them to gain physical and mental poise, improve their balance and give them a sense of accomplishment. Coordination is tied to balance and if children learn to balance then they can also improve on coordination. It can help children to gain mental clarity, stability, and increase their focus and attention naturally by them merely trying the poses. When a child learns to master a pose it can boost their confidence and self-esteem. They also help children to work various muscles in their bodies, strengthening, stretching and toning their bodies whilst enhancing their overall flexibility.

The names of postures are changed for children's yoga classes. Postures in a children's yoga class are more about how they feel in the body, rather than what they look like and proper alignment. Classes are intended to be fun and creative in naming poses. Changing the names of poses makes them more game like and can help to keep young children engaged and have fun. The creative names of poses are designed to let children play and use their imaginations. It also gives children an opportunity to connect with the pose and really be it.

Anyone participating in the class can make up names for poses, this gives opportunity for children to be creative and imaginative and for them to feel a part of creating a fun yoga class.

Lets take a look at some of the poses for a children's yoga class, a description of how to practise them and some of the amazing benefits they can bring.

SEATED POSTURES

Butterfly Pose, known as Baddha Konasana in Sanskrit. Sit on the sitting bones with the legs stretched out in front. Bend the knees and bring the soles of the feet together. Allow the knees to drop out to the sides. Sit tall and relax the shoulders. Open the feet with the hands as if the feet were a book. Finally fold forward over the legs and feet allowing the head to drop towards the feet. An alternative option in this posture is to take flight by sitting with the spine tall and flapping the knees up and down like wings.

Easy Seated Pose, known as Sukhasana in Sanskrit, translating to, posture or seat. This pose is performed by sitting in a simple crosss legged position and keeping the back straight and tall. The pose is often used for chanting, meditation and breathing. The posture brings stretching to the knees, it strengthens the back, opens up the hips and calms the mind. When regularly practising the easy seated pose, it is important to alternate the cross of the legs for a balanced stretching and strengthening of the body.

Flower Pose. Sit tall and hug the legs into the chest. Slide the elbows between and then under the knees. Lean back so that just the toes touch the ground. Lift the legs up, balance and breathe. Open the arms out like petals. Flower Pose develops the bodies core strength and balance.

Hero Pose, known as Virasana in Sanskrit. This pose can bring the feeling of being strong and confident.

To practise this pose, begin in the Japanese Sitting Pose, knees and shins on the floor whilst sitting on the heels, having a straight and tall back. This position brings a gentle stretch to the thighs, knees and ankles. Sitting in this way is also believed to help aid digestion. The blood flow is restricted to the lower half of the body, the legs and feet, and therefore more blood flow goes to the pelvic and stomach areas. More blood flow to the stomach area can aid in digestion and better bowel movement.

In Hero Pose the arms can be raised up over the head and actively stretched upwards. The fingers can be interlaced and palms turned over so that they face the ceiling. This movement helps to stretch and strengthen the back, shoulders and arms. Whilst in the position the sternum can even be expanded to bring feelings of a proud warrior. Children can then be guided to think about having a strong mind and body whilst in the pose. The pose can be held for around 30-60 seconds to begin with, or as long as is comfortable, and the duration can then be increased gradually.

River Pose also known as seated forward bend or Pashchimottanasana in Sanskrit. Sit with the legs straight out in front of the body. Press the hands down behind or by the sides of the body to lengthen the back. Then reach the hands towards the feet, hold onto the toes, shins or legs and stretch the chest out over the legs. The knees can be bent to help lengthen the spine whilst folding forward flowing like a river. Children can imagine that they are in warm water as they feel themselves melt with each breath.

Turtle Pose. Sit with the feet together and knees apart. Lift the arms then slide them under the knees. Place the hands on the floor outside of the feet. Round the back, reach the head towards the feet. Turtles have a safe, quiet space to go inside, the children can connect with this concept in this pose.

RESTING POSTURES

Childs Pose, known as Balasana in Sanskrit, meaning Bala - child, asana - pose, is a resting pose and can be used in a many beneficial ways in children's yoga. Childs Pose can also be known as, mouse, dormouse or rock pose.

To get into Childs Pose, sit comfortably on the heels with feet and knees together, arms by sides and back straight. Move the hands down to the floor and forward. Allow the belly, heart and forehead to come forward and rest the forehead on the ground between the hands. Observing the breath, feeling it moving in and out of the nose, feeling the belly and chest fill, pressing into the earth with the legs. Alternatively and for an even more restorative pose, the arms can be placed along the sides of the body with fingers towards the toes and palms facing up. Children can then be as quiet as a mouse.

This pose helps to stretch the hips, thighs and ankles. It gently relaxes the muscles on the front of the body whilst softly stretches the muscles of the back torso.

This resting pose centres, calms and soothes the brain, making it a therapeutic posture. Childs Pose restores balance and equanimity to the body. It can also be used as a counter pose to backbends.

It is a simple way to calm the mind, slow the breath and restore a feeling of peace and safety.

Polar Bear Pose is a resting and nurturing pose, similar in position and effect to Childs Pose. Polar Bear Pose is also a wonderful pose to spark the imagination and intertwine fun and learning topics into the yoga session.

Children can be guided to sit on their heels with their spine long and tall and head facing up. Make a V shape with the knees. Take a deep breath in and imagine that they are a big strong white polar bear. As they breath out to fold forward so that the chin touches the floor, or snow, the body should now be folded in-between the legs. Then bring the arms around so that the hands cup the chin. Continue breathing slowly and deeply and affirm that they are brave, quiet and relaxed.

The Polar Bear Pose can bring a sense of peace and relaxation to the whole body. It helps one feel grounded, secure and safe. The front organs in the body are massaged and it soothes the central nervous system as it gently lengthens and stretches the muscles along the spine and the hips. It is natural for children to go into this pose to relax, feel calm and to bring stillness to both their bodies and minds.

STANDING POSTURES

Aeroplane Pose. Stand with the feet parallel and under the hips. Breathe, focus and stretch one leg back. Tilt forward until the body is parallel with the floor. Spread the arms out like wings.

Dancers Pose, known as Natarajasana in Sanskrit. Stand tall in Mountain Pose. Bend the right knee bringing the right heel up towards the hips, hold the ankle with the right hand and lift the other arm up towards the sky. Bend forward and press the right leg into the hand up and backwards. Gently arch and extend the spine. If the children loose their balance just start again or find a friend or wall for support.

Dragon Pose. Stand on your knees, arms by sides. Lunge one foot forward, placing the hands on the thigh. Stretch the hips forward and down and reach the arms up. Exhale with a big, "Haaaa". Spread the fingers. Try breathing fire often to cleanse and strengthen the lungs.

Eagle Pose, known as Garudasana in Sanskrit. Cross the ankles. Cross the wrists and twist the thumbs down to interlace the fingers. Scoop the hands down and up to rest them at the heart. Breathe into the belly and remember someone or something you love.

Half Moon Pose, known as Ardha Chandrasana in Sanskrit. Stand with the legs apart, bend the right knee and step forward into a side lunge. Reach the right hand down to the floor under the shoulder. Extend the left leg parallel to the floor. Reach the left hand up. To come out of the pose, bend the standing leg, lower the raised foot and return to standing.

Mountain pose, known as, Tadasana in Sanskrit, is the foundation of all standing poses and brings awareness of how we stand. Mountain pose makes a great starting position, resting pose or a tool to improve posture.

Mountain Pose is all about learning to stand still, even for a few seconds, It is difficult for some children to keep their balance whilst standing still as it requirers the organisation of several senses by the brain and therefore promotes calm and mindfulness.

To practise Mountain Pose, stand tall with toes touching and feet slightly apart. If it is more comfortable, the feet can be further apart. Allow the body to gently sway back and forth and slowly bring the swaying to a standstill. Stop with weight balanced evenly on the feet. Press the shoulders back and straighten the arms beside the torso. Breathe deeply, and hold the pose for 30 to 60 seconds, or as long as is comfortable.

Practising balancing poses in yoga such as **Tree Pose**, can help gain physical and mental steadiness and poise. Tree Pose improves focus and coordination whilst calming the mind. The Sanskrit name for Tree Pose is, Vrksasana. Vrksa meaning tree and asana meaning pose.

Tree Pose with its calming and meditative benefits is like a standing variety of a seated mediative posture. Keeping calm and focused while balancing on one foot can teach children how to stay steady no matter what the outside circumstances may be.

Tree Pose stretches the thighs, groin, torso and shoulders. It improves the sense of balance and coordination. Regular practise will improve focus and ability to concentrate.

Due to the nature of Tree Pose being a balancing pose, it is important for students to practise the pose within their limits and ability. Adaptions to the pose can assist in helping students to work within their limits, holding onto a wall to begin with or resting the foot against the grounded foot to aid balance are options.

In order to fully gain the benefits of Tree Pose, it is important to stay grounded and calm in the pose. Working from the ground up can help with this. Starting with balancing the weight evenly on one foot grounding it into the earth like tree roots and then working up the legs, the trunk of the tree, the torso and extending through the crown of the head. Then placing the other foot on the inside of the standing leg, either resting the toes against the floor, on the inside of the calf or thigh. The arms and hands can be placed either in Anjali Mudra, palms together with thumbs resting at the heart space, or taking the arms above the head, palms together or arms apart for branches. Whilst holding the pose children can be asked what type of tree they are.

Triangle Pose, known as Utthita Trikonasana in Sanskrit. Step or jump the feet apart so that the feet are underneath the elbows if the arms are out to the sides. Turn the right foot out 90 degrees and the left foot in slightly. Lift the arms shoulder or just below the shoulder height. Tilt sideways over the right leg and stretch the arms wide. Lower the right hand to the right shin, ankle or floor trying to keep the body aligned as if between two walls.

Warrior Poses, known as, Virabhadrasana in Sanskrit, helps provide strength physically and mentally. Warrior 1 Pose can also evoke feelings of motivations and self respect. Affirmations relating to inner strength can be said whilst in the warrior poses, such as, "I believe in myself".

Physically ,Warrior 1 pose, improves balance and posture, stretches and strengthens the feet, ankles and calves and thigh muscles, improves mobility in the shoulder and hip joints and opens the chest and lungs.

To practise Warrior 1 Pose start in a high lunge. Turn the back heel down to the floor and press the feet down. Bring the hands to the leading thigh. Bend the front knee whilst reaching both arms up to the sky.

To practise Warrior 2 Pose, step or jump the feet apart. Turn the left foot in and the right foot out 90 degrees. Raise the arms out to the sides and stretch the arms away from each other. Turn the head to the right and bend the right knee. Try to keep the body weight in the centre of the pose.

ARM BALANCES & CORE STRENGTHENING POSTURES

Arrow Pose (Side Plank), Known as Vasisthasana in Sanskrit. Begin by being on the knees lifted up straight like an arrow. Extend the left leg out to the left side and place the right hand under the right shoulder, arm straight. Stretch the left arm up to the sky. Press down in the ground with the right hand and left foot lifting the hips up, slide right foot under left. To progress further into the pose, bend the left knee and lift the foot placing the sole on the inside of the right leg as if in Tree Pose. Use the tummy and leg muscles to balance. This pose requires confidence and a steady breath, a positive I can do mindset can be explored in this posture.

Boat Pose, known as Navasana in Sanskrit. Sitting tall with the knees bent, feet on the floor and taking the hands around the knees. Lean back taking the hands to the floor behind the back and point the toes. Engage the core from the belly. Lift up the legs feeling strong. Stretch out the arms in front of the body with the legs lifting, floating on the water like a boat. Hold for a few breaths.

Crow Pose. Squat with the feet together and knees open. Slide the backs of the upper arms under the knees. Lift the hips, press into the hands and shift the weight forward. Look forward, hug the knees and lift the feet up.

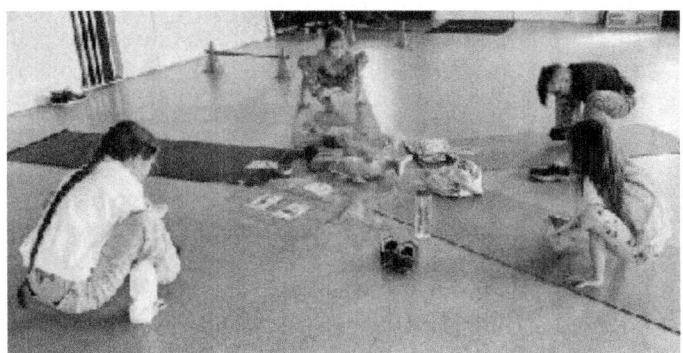

Arm balances are challenging. Playful determination can build strength, focus, balance and confidence. Children can imagine that their arms are crows legs and feet.

Dolphin Pose. Start on the knees and forearms with the toes curled under. Clasp the hands together. Push up on to the toes, lift the hips up to the sky and press the legs straight. Walk the feet in towards the elbows.

Plank Pose. Kneel on hands and knees. Shift the hands and body forward, chest and eyes lifted. Lower the hips so that the body is in a straight line. Curl the toes under, lift the core and straighten the legs. Build up strength by holding the pose for a little longer every day.

Scorpion Pose. Kneel, place the hands close together, fingers facing the feet. Tuck the elbows in so the upper arms support the torso. Lengthen the spine and legs, rest the forehead on the floor. Lift the feet, raise the head and chest and balance. Focus on the core and lengthening.

BACK BENDING POSTURES

The spine is an incredible combination of strength and flexibility. Strong bones and muscles give us structure and protect sensitive nerves while flexible ligaments and tendons allow the spine to move in all different planes. Practising back bends can help to protect this balance by increasing mobility while strengthening the supporting muscles around the skeleton.

Backbends are powerful poses and bring many benefits. As well as strengthening and increasing mobility they can elevate the mood by opening the heart and gently stimulating the nervous system. They can bring energy and help to relieve fatigue. Poses such as Mother Snake can stimulate the organs in the abdomen, improving digestion and open the chest bringing more oxygen into the lungs and heart. They can also improve circulation of blood and oxygen to the spine.

It is important that the body has warmed up before practising back bends and that appropriate poses are instructed to meet the students age and ability in a yoga class.

Bridge Pose, known as, Setu Bandha Sarvangasana, in Sanskrit, is a beginning backbend that helps to open the chest, improve flexibility in the spine and strengthens the core muscles. The Sanskrit name comes from five different words, Setu meaning bridge, Bandha meaning lock, Sarva meaning all, Anga meaning limb and Asana meaning pose. When in the full posture the arms and legs create a, locked bridge.

Because, Bridge Pose, opens the chest it increases the lung capacity and is therefore therapeutic to those with asthma. The pose also stimulates the abdominal organs and thyroid glands which can help improve digestion.

To practice Bridge Pose lie on the back with knees bent and feet on the floor, extend arms along the floor with palms facing down. Press the feet and arms firmly into the floor, exhale and lift the hips towards the ceiling. Draw the tailbone upwards and keep the buttocks off the floor. Roll the shoulders back and underneath the body. Keep the thighs and feet parallel and weight evenly across the feet. Hold for three or four breaths and slowly lower the hips.

A block or a blanket can be used under the lower back if needed to assist with raising the hips. It is recommended not to turn the neck left or right to prevent any neck injury. The pose should not be performed if a neck or shoulder injury is present.

Students can be encouraged to work on their own level of limits and ability and to be aware that these may feel different everyday. It is important to emphasise not to push the body to go deeper into the pose and that by relaxing in the pose the body will naturally open. The spine and shoulders and thighs tell how far to take the pose.

Camel Ride Pose, can help children prepare to practise the Camel Pose. Camel Ride Pose, is a more simpler pose than the Camel Pose. To practise the pose sit in the butterfly position, sitting on the bottom with legs bent and soles of feet together with back straight. Route the sitting bones into the ground and hold the ankles, breathe in and stretch the body forward, chest and stomach out. Breathe out and bring the chin towards the throat to open the spine, cave in the chest slumping the back and curving the spine. Using the pelvis, keep moving back and forth riding across the desert.

Camel Pose can be a challenging posture in yoga. The Camel Ride Pose can help prepare children's bodies for the Camel Pose by stretching and building strength to the spine. It can also help build confidence towards performing the camel pose in the future.

Practising the camel ride and camel pose can strengthen the back and shoulder muscles as well as help to reverse any forward rounding of the spine. It can bring fresh circulation that flows through the spine which will rejuvenate every system in the body as all systems are connected to the spinal cord. The rib cage is opened and stretched for good use of the lungs and digestive organs. In Arabian culture the camel symbolises patience, tolerance and endurance. Connecting to the camel can teach patience, determination and connection to the breath.

To practise Camel Pose, kneel with the knees hip width apart and toes curled under. Breathe as the spine is lengthened and shoulders broaden. Arch the chest, tilt the head to look up, extend the spine, roll the shoulders open and down and begin to drop backwards taking the hands to the feet. Squeeze the shoulder blades together and if comfortable allow the neck to relax back into the shoulder blades. Hold for 3-5 breaths, keeping the back of the neck long. To exit the pose, lead with the chest with the head coming up last. The toes can eventually be laid flat.

Cat Pose, known as Marjayasana is often paired with Cow Pose, known as Bitilasana. Cat Pose is a gentle forward bend and Cow Pose being a complimentary backward bend. Forward and backward bends feel very different physically and emotionally.

Backbends are energising and uplifting, whilst forward bends are contemplating and soothing and bring a quiet effect to the mind. They are opposites. One should follow a bend in one direction with a bend in the opposite direction to return the body to a state of balance.

To practise Cat and Cow Pose, start with being on the hands and knees, hands directly under the shoulders and knees under the hips. Point the fingertips to the top of the mat and stretch them like a cats paws. Place the shins and knees hip width apart. Centre the head in a neutral position and soften the gaze downward. Begin by moving into Cat Pose. Draw the belly into the spine and round the back towards the ceiling. The pose should look like a cat stretching its back. Release the crown of the head forward to the floor. Inhale and come into Cow Pose by dropping the belly forwards to the mat. Lift the chin and chest and gaze up toward the ceiling. Broaden across the shoulder blades and draw the shoulders away from the ears. This sequence can then be repeated.

This movement brings flexibility to the spine and can also help the body to become more coordinated.

Fish Pose, known as Matsyasana in Sanskrit. Sit up tall with legs straight. Lean back on the forearms. Lift the chest and arch the upper back and lean the head back so that the crown of the head rests against the floor. Breathe deeply as the pose is held for a few breaths. Yoga bricks can be useful for beginners to this pose by placing a block between the shoulder blades and one for the back of the head to rest on.

Grasshopper Pose, known as, Shalabasana in Sanskrit, is likened to that of a grasshopper or locust. The pose strengthens the muscles of the lower back area, gluteus and back of thighs.

To practise Grasshopper Pose, the children can be instructed to lie on their tummies with the legs together and straight resting on the floor. Bringing the hands together in front of the head with the elbows pointing out to the sides and the head resting on the hands. The tummy muscles can be tightened and whilst keeping the hips on the floor, one leg is raised a little off of the floor, stretching it behind. Then placing that leg down, the movement can be repeated on the other leg. Once completed the body can rest with arms down by the sides and head turned to one side. It is beneficial to turn the head to the other side during the rest to balance the gentle movement to the neck.

Following the Grasshopper Pose, a resting forward bend, such as Childs Pose, can be completed to ensure balance and energy to the body is neutralised.

Shark Pose. Lie on the tummy. Clasp the hands behind the back. Roll the shoulders back, lift the hands, feet and chest. Breathe, arch, lift and lengthen the whole body. Use this pose to develop strength, focus and determination.

Snake Pose and Mother Snake Pose are both backbends, the latter being the more challenging pose. Snake Pose is practised by lying on the floor on the tummy with legs straight and hands next to chest, palms down and the head and chest lifted. Mother Snake moves on from Snake Pose by pressing into the floor with the hands, straightening the arms and lifting the body up a little more, arching the spine but keeping the tummy on the floor. Children can hold Mother Snake for a few seconds then gently lower the back down to the starting position.

Follow Mother Snake with a neutralising pose such as Childs Pose. Whilst in the neutralising pose awareness can be bought to breathing into the back helping to cool down and relax the nervous system after the heat and energy created from a backbend.

Once a student is confident in the bridge pose it can be time to try the **Wheel Pose.** To execute this pose start in the same way as the bridge, instead of arms by the side extend the arms over the head and bend the elbows placing hands near the shoulders. Press down with the hands and feet to raise the body off of the floor while lifting the hips and chest towards the sky. A child can initially try to go onto the top of the head and then push up higher so that the full body is being held up by the hands and the feet. The easiest way out of the posture is by tucking the chin toward the chest and slowly lowering the body to the mat, one vertebra at a time.

Following the backward bend position of the wheel, neutralise the spine by bringing the knees up into the chest and taking the arms around them as if hugging them.

It is important to emphasise to students to listen to their bodies whilst practising these poses and only do what their body can do without any pain.

TWISTING POSTURES

Twists are a great way to squeeze out any frustrations. They also stimulate and detoxify the organs of the torso.

The **Lying Twist Pose**, is a great pose to help restore balance.

The Lying Twist Pose is practised by lying down on the back and hugging the knees to the chest. Breathing deeply in and out. Then breathe in and stretch the arms out on the floor at shoulder level or just below. Breathe out and let the knees fall slowly to the right, keeping one knee on top of the other. Slowly turn and look to the left with the head. Stay in the position for a few breaths, relaxing and feeling the back stretching. Whilst in the stretch children can imagine being a wet tee shirt with the water being wrung out of it. Breathe in and bring the head and knees back to the centre. Repeating the twist for the opposite side of the body.

The Lying Twist Pose offers many benefits. It stretches the back muscles and gluteus. It massages the back and hips. It helps to hydrate the spinal discs. It lengthens, relaxes and realigns the spine. It massages the abdominal organs and strengthens the abdominal muscles. The twist also encourages the flow of fresh blood to digestive organs, increasing health and function of the entire digestive system.

This pose is particularly beneficial and feels good after practising backbends. Lying Twist Pose is generally considered gentle and can be therapeutic. Students with any back pain or injury should approach this pose with caution as twisting the spine can make back pain worse.

Pretzel Pose a seated spinal twist known as Ardha Matsyendrasana in Sanskrit. Sit cross legged on the floor, lengthen the spine and connect the sitting bones with the earth. Bend the left leg over the right leg. Hook the right elbow outside of the left knee, left hand on the floor behind the body. Clasp the hands behind the back if the body allows. The children can imagine squeezing out all kinds of tension and be asked, what can they release. The children can also be asked to notice how they feel after the twist, are they more relaxed, open and alert.

INVERSIONS

Inversions, are asanas in yoga that take you upside down. The hips are higher than the heart and the heart higher than the head. Inversions are an integral part of a yoga practise. There are inversions at every level from Childs Pose to Headstand.

Inversions are mostly safe, however it depends on the person performing them. Some yoga teachers believe that children under 8 years of age, should not perform full inversions, this is to avoid any potential injuries to the neck muscles and joints and because of the strong effect they have on the thyroid gland, which for an adult can have a positive effect on the efficiency of the thyroid, however a child's thyroid should already be working at an efficient level.

There are huge benefits in practising inversions and a safe way to introduce them to children is through basic inverted postures where children are not putting any pressure on their necks or bodies. The following four poses are examples of basic inverted poses which are followed by advanced inversions.

Gorilla Pose, this pose is practised by standing with legs wide apart, bending forward from the waist and arms hanging loosely in front of the body. Once inverted swing the upper body from side to side like a gorilla. The children can even try to walk around on their big gorilla feet. For younger children they can stand up and beat the chest with the fists, making a loud gorilla sound. Gorilla pose brings the heart lower than the hips and higher than the head and benefits of inverted postures can be experienced.

The Standing Rag Doll Pose, as well as being a basic inversion, this pose also brings additional benefits of releasing tension in a controlled way by use of the breath and release of the body. To practise this pose, stand with the feet slightly apart, breathe in as the arms are lifted over the head and stretched. Breathe out in a big "aaaah" sound as the body flops forwards from the waist, releasing and letting the top half of the body be floppy and relaxed. To come out of the pose slowly come back up to standing.

Gorilla and Rag Doll Pose are also forward fold poses, that can be releasing and rejuvenating. The poses release and stretch the hips, hamstrings, calves and can stretch the entire backside of the body from head to heels.

Downward Dog pose is a good inverted pose to bring energy to the body. Inverted postures give the heart a rest. The heart works hard during the day, pumping oxygenated blood around the body, when inverted the blood flows more easily towards the upper part of the body, allowing the heart to take a break.

To practise downward dog start with the hands and knees on the floor, spread the hands and fingers and drop the head between the arms. Curl the toes under so that the balls of the feet are on the floor. Breathe slowly and smoothly as the legs are slowly straightened and lift the hips up into the air. Children can imagine that they are a dog stretching when they wake up from their nap. The pose can be held for three to four breaths and then the knees can be bought back down to the floor.

Practising Downward Dog pose also strengthens the arms and shoulders. It tones the core and waist area as the pose is held. It stretches the hamstrings and calves. It also lengthens the spine and back.

Precautions still need to be taken, for example warming up properly, listening to the body and progressing slowly are all good tips to consider. Ensuring that children do not hold such poses as downward dog for an extended period of time is also important as if not practised safely it could put pressure on their shoulders and wrists. Postures need to be approached carefully and mindfully.

Legs Up Position, this resting position can be one of the most nourishing, grounding and calming poses in yoga. The pose can also be easily used outside of the yoga class to help relieve feelings of being overwhelmed, tired or stressed.

To practise the pose, the back is flat on the floor with the sit bones as close to a wall as is comfortable. The legs are extended up the wall so that the backs of the legs are resting fully against it. For children the pose can be held for about ten breaths. To come out of the pose, bend the knees and roll over onto the side.

The position can help to relieve tired leg muscles and help drain tension from the legs and feet. The position can give the benefits of an inverted pose of reversing the effects of gravity on the whole body.

It is intended to be a deeply relaxing and a calming pose, especially when combining slow rhythmic breathing whilst in the pose. The body can feel safe and supported and this feeling can help reach a peaceful state.

Candle Pose is often referred to as the shoulder stand as the body weight rests on the top outer edges of the shoulders and the rest of the body lifts straight up into one line. This is an inversion that children can progress to. Ensuring the weight is on the shoulders prevents pressure being put on the delicate vertebrate of the neck. Blankets placed underneath the shoulders can help in keeping the neck free. It is important to not turn the head whilst in the pose and to look gently toward the chest to avoid injury to the neck. Directing the eyes toward the chest also keeps the pose calm and the neck soft.

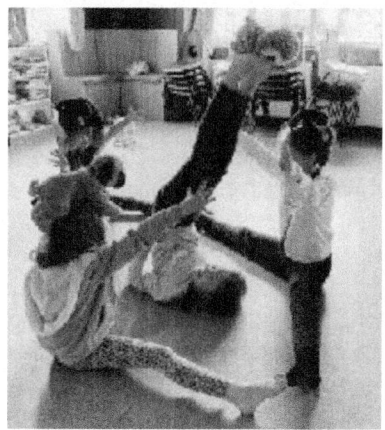

To practise Candle Pose, lie on the back, bring the knees up to the chest and wrap the arms around them, rock backwards and forwards a few times, then slowly lift the legs, lower back and hips into the air. Put the hands on the lower back palms facing in towards the body. Push the body up so that the body weight is resting on the shoulders. Breathe comfortably. When ready to come down, roll out slowly, bringing the back down first then the legs. The time the pose is held can be gradually built up. After practising the Candle Pose it is advisable to rest on the back for a few moments.

Variations for beginners to the pose, can use a wall for support. Pressing both feet into the wall with knees bent, this action takes some weight off of the shoulders and helps make alignment of the body easier. Progression from this variation can be to then lift one foot off of the wall and straightening the leg holding and then returning the foot to the wall, repeat with the other leg.

Handstand. Many children love to practise handstand and you may find some of your students already practise this fun pose outside of yoga. This is another inversion that children can work towards by building the strength in their arms, shoulders and core. Using the wall to help learn a controlled handstand is a great way to start.

To practise the first steps of handstand, sit with the back against the wall with legs straight, place two yoga bricks to mark the distance the feet are away from the wall. This is where the hands will go. Then moving to all fours, place the hands in line with the bricks and begin to walk the feet up the wall so that the feet come to a 90 degree angle, hold the pose for a few breaths or as long as comfortable and then walk the feet back down. Resting in Childs Pose for a few breaths. This pose can then be progressed by continuing to use the wall for support by placing the hands close to the wall in Downward Facing Dog and then walking the feet in towards the face, bending one knee and then pushing up the other straight leg into a handstand, having the wall behind the body for support if needed. Whilst holding the pose push down with the hands into the floor, looking between the hands, engage the core, bringing the feet and legs together. Once confident in this pose children can then practise without the wall.

Snail Pose, known as Halasana in Sanskrit. Snail pose can be a challenging pose for some people and is another inversion that children can work towards. To practise Snail Pose lie on the back, bring the knees up to the chest and wrap the arms around them, rock backwards and forwards a few times, then slowly lift the legs, lower back and hips into the air. Bring the hands on the lower back palms facing inwards. Gently bring the legs over the head and allow the feet to drop towards the floor resting the toes against the floor. A cushion or other prop can be used to rest the feet upon if they don't reach the floor. As an option the knees can be bent, relaxing the legs and allowing the knees to come towards or rest on the floor next to the ears. When ready to come out of the pose, roll out slowly, bringing the back down first then the legs. The time the pose is held can be gradually built up. After practising Snail Pose it is advisable to rest on the back for a few moments. Whilst in Snail Pose children can be reminded that they have everything they need within themselves and they can rest in their shell.

CREATIVE WAYS TO INTRODUCE ASANAS

Introducing yoga postures into the asana part of the class can be done in many different ways. A teacher can lead postures using a story, or take inspiration from yoga cards or by means of fun and creative games.
Here are some fun ideas on how to introduce the asana part of the class.

Animal Yoga Cards
Gather images, drawings or yoga cards of animals that match a theme. Place them face up for children to choose their favourite for the asana part of the class. Provide information and discussion about the animals whilst holding the postures.

Animal Bag
Put together a bag of wooden animals. Each child takes a turn to pick an animal out of the bag. Be creative and make up a pose or practise a yoga pose that matches that animal.

Beachball
Write or draw poses onto a beachball. Take turns to throw the ball to a friend, the child that catches the beachball, wherever their right thumb lands, everybody takes that pose. This is a great game for an ocean, water or beach themed yoga class and the poses can be related to the topic.

Charades
Place yoga cards face down, each child picks a card. Each player then takes turn to perform the pose, others guess what they are. A correct guess gives the guesser the next go, ensure all children have a go.

Choose your Pose
Choose three yoga poses. Leader turns back and everyone chooses one of the three poses to hold. Leader calls out a pose and then turns around. Everyone holding that pose wins and gets to stay in the game, everyone else sits down. Leader again calls out a pose and then turns back around to face the group. Play continues until there is a winner.

Circus Skills
Appoint a Ringmaster, this child names acts from a circus such as a juggler, acrobat, clown the children can either create their own Yoga Pose to represent the act or poses can be assigned to acts. Try to allow each child a turn at being the Ringmaster.

Dice Yoga Pose
This is a simple way to introduce yoga poses, roll the dice, and perform the yoga pose matching the number rolled.

Discover an Animal Friend
In ancient times the concept of power animals being magical helpers for individuals was rooted in the bones of many people. Sit cross legged or in a comfortable position. Close the eyes. Focus on the breathing in and out through the nose. Ask yourself what animal do you feel most drawn too or connected with. Share your animal friend with the group. Match or make up a pose for your animal friend. If children don't have one pick an animal yoga pose card.

Grateful Asanas
Place Nature themed yoga cards for the children to see. Invite each child to pick a card that they like. Practise each pose as a group and ask the child who picked the pose what they are thankful for about their nature item, e.g thank you for the oxygen given by the trees.

Invent a Pose
Begin with a bag of stuffed or wooden animals. Each child takes a turn drawing an animal out of the bag. Think of a pose that would resemble the animal. Be the teacher and teach that pose to the rest of the class.

Lucky Dip Yoga Pose
Children pick a Yoga card or toy out of a bag or box, perform the pose showing how to practise it, teach the other children how to do the pose.

Mantra Magic & Positive Affirmations
Use Yoga Cards that have a matching mantra. Have everyone pick out a favourite pose from the yoga cards and use the given mantra or affirmation or make up your own. Have everyone share what their chosen mantra means to them and when they may need to use it. In a circle everyone takes a turn making their pose and saying their mantra or affirmation with confidence. Continue around the circle.

Magical Yoga Stories
Select Yoga pose cards that inspire the imagination for a story. Lay the cards out in the middle of the room and invite the children to choose their favourite. The children will create a story using their pose, each taking a turn to add their part of the story. Practise the poses as the story is made. Put on a yoga play once you have your story.

Match Yoga Poses
Provide a selection of yoga cards and allow the children to choose one. Play music and invite the children to move or dance around the room. When the music stops, call out instruction such as. Find a partner with an opposite

pose, or a pose that flows together, then practise both poses together. Repeat giving opportunity for children to find a new partner.

Memory Yoga Game
Choose a child to start, this child performs a yoga pose, the next child practises the first child pose and then adds another, play continues.

Mini Olympic Games
Mini games course, set up the mats in a large rectangle or circle shape, on each mat place Yoga cards or instructions for an olympic games course. The children then complete the course. For example wind surfer - Warrior 2, gymnastics - Dancer pose, horse riding - Chair pose, rowing - Boat pose. You can also use exercises that warm up the body or are just fun that aren't Yoga poses such as cycling - lying on the back lifting the legs and cycling the legs, or swimming - lying on the tummy pretending to swim.

Musical Yoga Dots
Place a yoga cards under dots around the room, play music and direct children to move or dance around the room. When the music stops find a dot and Yoga card and hold the pose.

Musical Mats
Using Yoga cards practise poses. Then place one Yoga card on each mat. Play some fun music, the children can move or dance around the mats, when the music stops find a mat and perform the pose that is on the mat.

Nature Yoga Cards
Gather images, drawings or yoga cards of nature that match the theme and season. Place them face up for children to choose their favourite for the asana part of the class. Provide information and discussion about nature whilst holding the postures.

Operation
Use operation game to be surgeons, each child takes a turn to choose a body part from the game to remove and then practise a yoga pose that helps that part of body.

Opposites
Using yoga cards, pick a card and try to come up with an opposite pose. e.g Downward Facing Dog pose could become Boat Pose.

Pick a Yoga Card
Each child takes a turn to pick a Yoga card, all children practise pose. Taking this further, ask the children to create a flow of the poses using the cards, play some music and practise the flow.

Popstick Yoga
Start by writing or drawing a favourite yoga pose on craft sticks, place each stick in a jar. Let the children pick a craft stick, and perform the yoga pose written or drawn on the stick. The poses can relate to a theme of the class.

Put on Diving Gear
Go explore the ocean. Begin by pretending to put on diving equipment. Dive into the water and swim around the ocean. You can only use hand signals now to point things out. Place ocean themed yoga pose cards around the room and direct the children to swim to find their favourite ocean animal. Then return to the yoga mats and remove the diving equipment. Talk about what animals the children picked and practise the pose. Some ocean themed Yoga poses are whale, dolphin, crab, fish, shark, jellyfish, mermaid, octopus, turtle, star fish.

Ring Around the Yogi (age 2-5)
Ring around the Yogi is sung to Ring around the roses. Ring around the Yogi, Ring around the Yogi, tree pose, tree pose, we all fall down. Different poses can be used to replace tree pose.

Strike a Pose
Place the pose cards facedown in a pile. Take turns flipping over the top card and everyone has to strike the pose as fast as they can.

Time to Shine
Children perform favourite pose/move/anything to group. Each child can also teach the other children their pose or move.

Twister
Spread out yoga cards and group them according to different body parts that will be touching the ground, e.g two hands and two feet poses for these body parts could be Downward Facing Dog Pose or Plank Pose. Two feet no hands instructions could be Warrior 1 or 2 or Mountain Pose. Once the cards are sorted into groups, call out different hand/feet/back combinations.

Wendy Witch
Like Simon Says game, use Wendy Witch says, then instruct a Yoga pose, the last child into the pose gets turned into a black cat.

Yoga Assault Course
Set up the mats in a large rectangle or circle shape, on each mat place Yoga cards or instructions for an assault course. The children then complete the course. You can also additional props for each mat such a bean bags, skip

ropes, yoga bricks as a beam, egg & spoon for balance. Having a mindfulness mat at the end is a good addition to any assault course.

Yoga Bingo
Yoga bingo cards. Place yoga pose cards face down and take turns picking a card. Make Yoga bingo cards with poses that match the cards. Any players who have the pose picked on their card can demonstrate the pose and mark the space on their card. Game can continue until there is a winner.

Yoga Flow
While sitting in a circle, everyone selects a yoga pose card and demonstrates one at a time how to make that pose. Continue around the circle with everyone demonstrating their chosen pose. Play some music whilst all the children holds each child's pose for a few rounds of breath. Continue around the circle.

Yoga Jenga
Write or draw yoga poses on the Jenga blocks. Play Jenga, perform the Yoga pose writing on the block pulled out. Game continues until the tower falls down.

Yoga Pictures
Organise the children into two teams. Both teams choose a member to be the drawer. Ever drawer selects the same pose card. They then draw the pose. Each team tries to guess the name of the pose. When guessed everyone on that team demonstrates it.

Yoga Plays
Pick 3 or 4 Yoga poses from Yoga cards. Practise the poses together. Then give the children some time to be creative to make a story, a scene or a poem using the Yoga poses. Perform to the other group or groups.

Yoga Pose Challenge
Give different instructions of body parts that can touch the floor, for example 1 foot, 1 foot and one hand, the back. Children then enter into a Yoga pose with just the body parts given touching the floor.

Yoga Queen or King
Select a yoga queen or king. They are in command and get to dictate to his or her subjects the yoga poses performed. They call out a yoga pose and everyone must hold the pose. The king or queen walks around and inspects everyones pose and crowns a new ruler.

Yoga Spinner Game

Each child takes a turn to spin a spinner, practise the Yoga Pose the spinner lands on. Keep going until someone has collected 2 or 3 cards.

SEQUENCING

Practising one pose at a time is good for building body strength and flexibility and it can help children focus on their alignment. Children can learn more about body anatomy and awareness of their bodies when doing yoga poses one at a time. Practising this way can also teach children about patience and stamina.

Sometimes however, children may need to go through yoga poses more quickly to really get them moving and feeling active. They may need to burn off energy or raise the heart rate to help them wake up and stay focused. Moving children through poses faster can help to keep them focused.

A yoga sequence is a specific set of yoga poses practised in a row, and when repeated, usually in the same order. Yoga sequencing can be done slowly with breaks in between, or more quickly.

Sequences can be predetermined based on, the energy need of the children, a particular theme or story and children can also create their own sequences.

Most sequences are one posture following another in a logical step by step direction, mainly from less challenging to more challenging and back to less challenging. Typically each posture is performed once but can be practised two or three times focusing on a different aspect of the posture each time.

PARTNER & GROUP WORK

Mastering the art of being a team player will help children throughout their lives. Getting along and engaging with others is the building block of many things in life. From a young age children learn how to give and take, share and take turns, this being a core social skill. It is important for children to also learn to build relationships, whether with family members, friends or others.

Learning to work in a partnership or a group will help children hone many social skills, such as patience, empathy, communication, respect for others, compromise and tolerance. It can also help develop confidence in themselves and trust in other people.

It is quite normal for some children to have difficulty at first with partner and group work. They can be the centre of their own world and their needs come first. It can be hard for them to put those aside to allow someone else's needs to be met. Overtime children can get used to being part of a group and are able to do some give and take, share with others, and show empathy towards other children.

Yoga can give excellent opportunities for children to work in partnership with each other and can cultivate a team work ethos that children can draw on throughout their life.

During partner of group work, it is important to encourage children to change partners and groups regularly so that they can get to know everyone in the group. This practise also promotes a respect for others by taking time to get to know everyone in the group, inclusiveness of all and also offers opportunity for new experiences with a different partner or group.

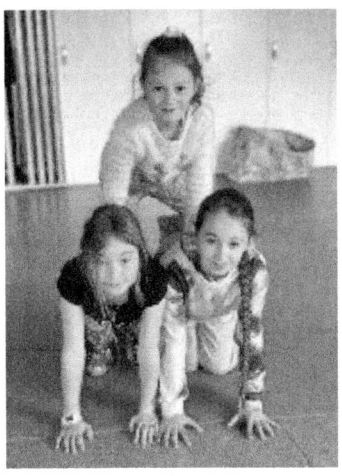
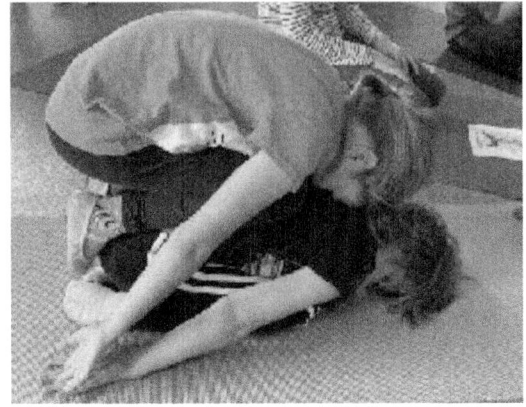

IDEAS FOR PARTNER AND GROUP WORK

Balance Poses
Choose a selection of balancing poses to practise together. Children can support each other if they need some help for balance.

Beachball Pass
Sitting in a group pass a beach ball around the group. Using hands above head, twist to the side, stretch forward, then use feet and legs.

Cant Move Me
Choose a partner of similar height, choose an anchor and lifter. Lifter places arms around the waist of their partner and lifts them off the ground. Then anchor stands feet apart and imagines being anchored and immobile by sending energy down into the earth like roots of a tree. Lifter repeats the lift of their partner again. Being able to ground the self makes it much harder or impossible to be lifted. This practise connects children with earths stable and strong energy.

Community Circle
Sitting in a circle give one child a ball and invite that child to roll or throw that ball to a friend saying something that they appreciate about that person, helping to lift each other up.

Dog or Animal Chase
Use two soft toys, sit in circle, pass toys around using feet until the chaser catches the runner, (dog and cat).

Downward Facing Dog Tunnel
Children perform Downward Facing Dog Pose next to each other creating a tunnel. The child at the start of the tunnel goes down onto their stomach and crawls through the tunnel. Once at the end of the tunnel that child joins the tunnel and the next child takes a turn. Repeat until all children have crawled through the tunnel.

Gratitude Meditation
Sit in a comfortable position where your spine can be tall and your shoulders relaxed. Close your eyes for this short meditation. Take a few relaxed calming breaths in and out through the nose. Notice how your body feels and your feelings when you breath this way. (pause)
Imagine the things for which you are grateful for. (pause)
Think of the people for which you are thankful. (pause).
Bring your focus back to your breath and your body.
When you are ready open your eyes.

Group Massage
Children to sit in a circle facing each others back. Using fingertips gently massage each others neck, shoulders, arms and back. Think about how it feels when we give to others and also when we receive from others.

Group Yoga Pose Flow
Using the yoga postures practised in the asana section of the class. Allow the children to create a flow of the postures by putting them in a certain order. Play music and practise the yoga flow together, holding each pose for a few breaths before flowing into the next posture.

Love it or Leave it
Call out random items, such as chocolate, water, apples, maths, nature, dogs, cats etc,,,. If children love it they stand up on their toes and balance with their arms open, if children leave it they go into Childs Pose.

Make Nature Scenes
As a group or in partners, holding a Yoga Pose or shape with the body, make a group nature scene, such as from a rainforest or ocean themed Yoga class.

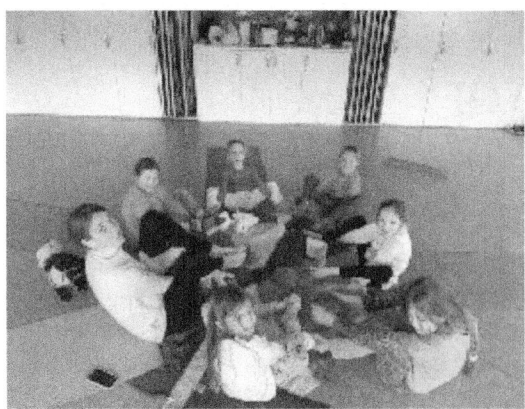

Make Structures
As a group or in partners, holding a Yoga Pose or shape with the body, make structures such as the Eiffel Tower, a bridge, boat etc…

Partner Poses
Using partner pose Yoga cards, see if partners can complete all the partner yoga cards . Then create a new pose together. Come up with a name and demonstrate it to the group.

Partner Volcano Pose
Stand facing each other approximately arms lengths apart, invite the children to repeat."We are partners". Press each others palms together and move so that the arms are straight whilst palms together. State, "We touch our palms". Lean towards each other and raise hands upwards whilst stating, "We press up". Pushing the hands up and together as high as can whilst stating, "We hold each other up".

Partner Yoga Pose Practise
Each child takes a partner Yoga card. The children walk around to find someone who has the same colour shirt (or eyes, top, shoes, etc). Once everyone is matched up, the partners practice the poses on their cards together

Plough Race
Have the children sit up tall with legs straight in front one behind the other. The first child begins with a ball between their feet. They roll up into Snail Pose and pass the ball to the child sitting behind them, using their feet only. The second child takes the ball with their feet and repeats until the last child receives the ball.

Rainbow Power
Stand face to face with a friend and move several feet apart. Imagine you are a rainbow and feel how beautiful you are. Now, just like sending a message, send your rainbow to your friend. Then, ask him/her to describe how it felt. Invite him/her to send you a rainbow. Tell him/her how it felt.

Rock Tree Bridge
As a group, the first child makes a rock in Childs Pose, the 2nd child jumps over the rock and makes a Tree Pose, the 3rd child jumps over the rock, runs around the tree and makes a Bridge Pose, the 4th child then begins to repeat the pattern of rock tree bridge.

Surfboard Competition
Play cool surfing style music such as The Beach Boys Surfing USA. Invite the children to pretend that they are surfing on their mats, when the music stops hold a pose practised in the class.

Tea Party
As a group make a table and chairs together. Enjoy a tea party.

Tree Community
Practise Tree Pose as a group, a community. Make a big circle and support each other in Tree Pose. Try different ways to do this, standing, lying on the

floor. You can develop this further by making different shapes and creating human mandalas.

Trick or Treat
Set up a few stations around the room for makeshift doors to knock on for trick or treat. Have a yoga card at the stations for the children to do poses. They can also receive a treat for the demonstration of their pose.

Trust Game
Working in partners, choose one child to close their eyes and the other child to lead their partner around an assault course. Use props and equipments to make a course such as skipping ropes, yoga bricks, bean bags etc….

Wash Away
Think of something you want to let go of…imagine it washing out. Stand with your arms hanging. Twist from your hips so your arms swing out and wrap around you, first one way, then the other. Repeat until you feel clean and clear.
Think of something you want more of…imagine tapping it in. Start at the top of your head. Tap down your front to your toes, then tap up the back of your body from your heels to your head. Tap across both your shoulders and down and up your arms. Repeat until you feel refreshed.
You can always wash out what weighs you down and tap in to what lightens you up!

Yoga Poetry
Working in small groups and using the yoga poses practised in the asana section of the class, give the children direction to create a short story or poem connecting with the theme of the class. Perform to the other group or groups.

RELAXATION

Relaxation, known as, Shavasana in yoga, is one of the most challenging and powerful poses. Being still is not easy and takes practise. Even if a struggle at the beginning, there are still many benefits. Practising relaxation can calm the mind, relieve stress, bring physical relaxation, reduce fatigue and promote sleep.

A way to introduce children to relaxation is through a regular yoga class where the children can become familiar with other children in the group, the yoga teacher and the basic structure of the class. Relaxation can start simply to begin with. A good introduction to relaxation for children is to start with something that they are familiar with, like sleep.

By relating to something children already know about, like sleep, the brain can develop from the knowledge already stored about the subject and can build on this knowledge to learn new things quicker.

Children can be asked to think about which position is most comfortable for them to relax in and to lie down on the floor in that position. Children can then be asked what position they lie in before they go to sleep at night and to move around until they find their most relaxing position. They can then be instructed to close their eyes and pretend to go to sleep. This relaxation can be practised for a short amount of time to begin with, one or two minutes.

Once children are more familiar with relaxation, relaxation techniques can be developed, and children can obtain skills to practise relaxation and mindfulness from an early age.

Taking time to relax is really important in maintaining positive mental health. There are many techniques and ideas that can help children relax deeper and learn to enjoy relaxation.

Moving the body before relaxation and being able to express oneself during activities in a yoga class can help lead to a child being able to relax with more ease.

Controlled breathing will promote calm and helps the body relax and releases muscle tension. Using the breath is a great way of encouraging children to relax. A fun technique to use controlled breathing is to have children lie their heads on the belly of the friend next to them. The children can be asked to breath deeply and feel how they lift and lower their friends head with their body and also how the same happens to their head. Eyes can be closed and a focus on listening and feeling the breath may help children go into a deeper relaxation.

Using counting during relaxation can also help children relax. Asking the children to sit or lie in a comfortable position, close their eyes and count 10 to 20 breaths can help calm the mind and aid in the experience of relaxation.

Some children may need to move and feel secure during a relaxation and the sitting rag doll pose can help. Sitting on the floor with legs out in front with arms by sides, the arms can then be stretched out and up to be as tall as possible. The child can imagine that they are a soft and floppy rag doll and can bend forwards to let the upper body rest on the legs. The arms can flop loosely on the floor. The child can then return slowly to sitting back up.

To help children become aware of their bodies and relax them a relaxation technique of naming body parts can also be practised. This technique is based on the traditional practise of Shavayatra a relaxing technique of naming parts of the body in order and to sense that part of the body and move on. A fun way to do this with children is to ask the children to pretend their bodies are like spaghetti. Start by asking the children to lie down on their backs and make their bodies really stiff like uncooked spaghetti. Then ask what happens if the spaghetti is cooked, suggesting that it becomes soft and flexible and can move in any direction. The children can be directed that thats what their legs, arms and body can do to be able to relax. This exercise can teach children what relaxation feels like in their bodies.

Props can also be used to help children relax. A small stone or pebble can be placed on the forehead. This can be a special yoga magic stone or pebble that they can imagine gives magic powers, for example, powers of talking to animals, or powers of flying. The stone or pebble needs to stay on the forehead, if it falls off the powers stop. This technique can help children stay still and relax and receive the benefits.

Tibetan Singing Bowls are another special prop that can be used to help children relax and focus their attention. The sound of the singing bowl is believed to also bring healing. A way to use the bowl could be to visit each child whilst they are lying on their backs, place the bowl on their chest or belly and gently tap the bowl so that the children feel the sound and vibration.

Props that help bring a cosy and secure feeling can also be used to help relaxation. Cushions or blankets can be used to make a cosy den for the children to relax together. Blankets can give extra weight on the body which can help children to be less fidgety. Yoga mats can be used to wrap themselves up like an Egyptian mummy, helping children to feel secure and protected for relaxation.

All of these techniques and many others can help children be introduced and experience relaxation in a fun and focused way. A relaxed child is able to think more positively and gives them space to step back and reflect. Learning how to relax and allowing relaxation in ones life, is a vital life skill that can bring good health and well being.

One of the most powerful, yet simple, self-awareness tools is guided imagery. It uses words and images to help move the attention away from worry, stress and pain to help find inner strength and creativity. This brings the natural powers of the mind into health and healing.

Through guided imagery the imagination can create a particular state of emotion, it can actually change feelings by changing the focus. Even very young children can learn this skill by linking images in their minds with feelings and experiences.

Guided imagery can have many health-related physical and emotional benefits. It can lessen feelings of being nervous or upset, help with pain management or achieve a goal such as an athletic or academic achievement.

The mind is a very powerful tool that can have a tremendous effect on the body. The body reacts the same whether we are actually experiencing something or just imagining something.

Imagery can have a positive effect on heart rate, blood pressure, breathing and oxygen rates, brain waves, temperature, and hormone balance. Guided imagery can help relieve symptoms caused or made worse by stress, such as headaches and digestive and breathing problems.

At the end of a guided visualisation in yoga it is important to allow children to process the visualisation and to slowly bring the guided imagery to an end. Ending the visualisation and getting the children to then breathe in and out deeply and open their eyes aims to bring their experience of that imagery to a close and to bring their awareness back to the present moment and environment. Having the children follow some physical movements, like clapping their hands 10 times, rubbing their hands together to warm them and place them on their face, rubbing the head and hair, the back of the neck, placing their hands over their ears and then slowly standing up. These movements should bring a child's awareness back to their own physical body and their physical presence in the yoga class.

All of these benefits can tie together and help children learn to accept and love themselves and others. It can help them focus and calm their minds and they can learn tools to help them be resilient. They are more likely to be positive about life and their ability and less likely to suffer anxiety and other mental health issues. It can show children that relaxation is allowed and encouraged in their life.

Here are some examples of guided relaxations -

All is Well
Rest back and relax. Close your eyes and go inside. Breathe and know that all is well. Repeat softly or silently, "May I be safe and loved. May I be happy and healthy. May I be kind and caring. May I know that all is well."

Animal Friend
Settle down and relax. Close your eyes and go inside. Breath in love and breathe out worry. Imagine you are outside. The sun is shining, birds are singing. You hear a rustling in the bushes and then a giggle. Its an animal watching you and it wants to be your friend. What kind of animal is it? Let it come close so that you can sit together and be close. This animal is wise and here to support you. If you have a question, or a problem you can share it with him. He will help you. Your animal friend loves you very much.

Autumn
Imagine you are outside in the beautiful autumn air. Pretend for a moment that you are the wind. You glide peacefully along the sunny pleasant day. The air smells fresh all around you. As you glide you pick up some leaves along the way. How wonderful to feel the connection to these beautiful autumn leaves. Sometimes you are strong, and other times you are very gentle. Feel your gentle strength as you calmly blow across the tress and rich earth. And now imagine changing into a leaf floating on the wind. Feel yourself as a beautiful soft leaf dancing in the wind so gracefully. You are letting the wind carry you where it wants. Now you start to drift back down to earth, back down to your mat, becoming yourself once more. You can open your eyes when you are ready.

Beach Relaxation
Lie back, close your eyes and breathe slowly and deeply. Imagine lying on a beach, the sand is soft and comfy. The sun is warm. Feel a gentle breeze. Relax your whole body, feel your head and face nice and cool and relaxed. Feel your head, neck, chest, arms and hands relaxed. Feel your tummy moving up and down warm and relaxed. Feel your back, legs, feet and toes warm, relaxed and heavy. Feel warm and comfortable and at peace. Relax with this comfortable feeling for a few moments more.
Breathe in and bring some gentle movement to the body, become aware of the room around you, the yoga mat underneath you, and bring some movement back to the body. When you are ready open the eyes.

Be a Rainbow
Relax and close your eyes and go inside. Slow down your breathing, sigh ahhh. Let go and melt into the floor. Imagine you are walking down a beautiful path. A storm is leaving and you see a rainbow. Stand under it and let its warm, bright light fill you with happiness. You are connected to all life. You are a rainbow too. Red you are strong and safe, orange you are happy and playful, yellow you are proud and confident, green you are kind and caring, blue you are honest and truthful, indigo you are clever and creative, violet you are a good friend.

Body Awareness
Lie back. Make your body stiff like uncooked spaghetti. Then imagine your body turns into soft and loose cooked spaghetti. Next place your hands on your soft tummy, can you feel your breath? Place your hands on your chest, can you feel your breath, your heart beating? Can you feel your back of your body resting on the floor, the back of your head, your shoulders, your hips, legs and feet. Relax here for a few more breaths.

Colour Meditation
Imagine any colour. Notice what it is like, light, dark? See yourself surrounded by a big bubble. Imagine the colour spreading over you colouring you. As you lie still, feel the colour all around you.
When ready slowly open the eyes and notice how you feel.

Flower Garden
Lie down in a comfortable position and allow your body to become heavy and relaxed. Allow your tummy to fill up like a balloon and then exhale slowly. Do this three times to really relax your whole body. As your body relaxes, imagine you are a beautiful butterfly fluttering high in the sky. You see the lovely green fields below you with lots of colourful flowers just waiting for you to enjoy. You feel the wind blow against your delicate wings. As the wind touches you, it gently blows away any worries you may feel. Feel how wonderful it is to be free. Your mind is clear and calm.
You are completely peaceful. You are beautiful as you allow your true happiness to shine through.
The earth below you is a patchwork of colour and you enjoy each moment here, gliding along feeling so joyful and peaceful. You can fly around as long as you like, exploring or just floating gently on the wind. (pause).
Take in a deep breath now and exhale slowly. Give your body a big stretch to awaken. Open your eyes and take in the surroundings of the room feeling peaceful and calm ready for the rest of your day.

Guiding Star
Imagine you are outside at night. You look up and notice one very bright star. It sends a light beam down directly to you. Breathe in its warmth and

wonder. You feel yourself glow. Now the star is moving. Follow and find out what the guiding star is leading you to. It is a message for you, do what lights you up and let yourself shine.

Inner Light
Lie in a comfortable position, relax your body and close your eyes. Imagine now a small sparkle somewhere deep inside your heart. The small sparkle begins to glow brighter. The glow becomes brighter and brighter filling up your chest. You feel the warmth spreading out touching your tummy, your shoulders, getting bigger and bigger. Getting brighter and brighter glowing all the way to your toes. Now feel your whole body glowing like a radiant star shining out. This wonderful light is your light. Shine your light wherever you go.

Lantern Meditation
Settle down and relax, close your eyes. Imagine seeing a lantern being lighted for you, as you do this, think about something you are ready to let go of. It could be an event that happened, something you are ready to free your mind from thinking about. Try to notice what did this experience teach you. Your lantern is filling with hot air, knowing it is time to fly, release the lantern. Now think of something you would like, something to experience, enjoy or to try. What do you invite into your life. Holding this intention like a light in your heart, breath in, feeding the light with oxygen, exhale, release your intention into the Universe like a lantern.

Loving Guided Meditation
Lie in a comfortable position, relax your body and close your eyes.
Imagine that you are sending love to yourself, send yourself a message that says, "I love you". Now tell your body that you love it, notice how your body feels when you tell it that. Now think of someone in your family or a good friend, send them some love. Now think of all the people all over the world, send them some love too. Now imagine all of these people you've sent love to and imagine that each of these people sends love back to you. Feel their love coming back to you.

Peace Relaxation
Lie down and close your eyes. Imagine your belly is like the ocean. With each inhale the waves rise and with each exhale they fall. Feel your belly rising and falling as you breathe. Now imagine there is a small boat on your ocean. What does it look like? You want to help guide the boat toward the shore. You can do this by taking nice slow deep breaths in and out through your nose. Create a steady rhythm for your boat. As your belly rises and falls, continue to guide your boat. After a few cycles of slow and steady breathing imagine your boat has safely landed on the shore. Now bring your attention back to the rise and fall of your belly as you breath in and out.

Begin to notice how you feel, is your breathing different does your body feel different? What about your mind? Now say something kind to yourself. You are wonderful, you are special, you are peace. When you are ready gently bring yourself to a seated position.

Positive Thoughts
Find a comfortable position. Relax your body and feel the support of the floor beneath you. Close your eyes. Take some relaxed breaths in and out through the nose.
Begin to create a picture in your mind, imagine a place where you feel completely at ease. This might be a favourite place, somewhere you've been or it might be completely imaginary. Picture this place where you feel happy and calm. Enjoy the way you feel in this place, rest in this place.
Imagine these affirmations to build self esteem are true for you.
I am at peace with myself. I accept myself. I deserve to be happy. I feel confident. I am perfectly alright just the way I am.
Now its time to leave your special place, know that you can return here in your imagination anytime to relax and feel calm. Take with you the feelings and beliefs in yourself.
Begin to move and awaken your body. Stretch. Roll to one side and come to seated.

Radiant Start
Gently close your eyes and relax. Allow your body to sink down into the Earth. Allow the muscles to become soft and relaxed. Imagine now a small sparkle somewhere deep inside your heart. The small sparkle begins to glow brighter and brighter filling up your chest. You feel the warmth spreading out touching your tummy and shoulders. Getting brighter and brighter, glowing all the way to your toes. Now let your whole body glow like a radiant star, shining out. This wonderful light is your light, shine your light wherever you go.

Springtime
Lie down in a comfortable position and allow your body to become heavy and relaxed. Close your eyes and notice how your breath flows in and out of your body. Imagine breathing in peacefulness and breathing out any tension so that you feel calm and relaxed.
Imagine yourself walking outdoors, the sun shines down warmly on you.
You see a beautiful meadow, it would be so nice to sit down in the grass.
Find a place to sit or lie down. Feel the breeze on your skin.
Notice the sights around you, the grass, wildflowers, butterflies around you. Rest in this peaceful, beautiful meadow. (pause)
Now it is time to leave the meadow and return to this moment.

Feel the floor beneath you, hear the sounds of the room and open your eyes and see the room around you. Take a moment to stretch your body and allow yourself to reawaken.

Special Place
Sit back and relax. Breathe deeply and slowly. Close your eyes and go inside. Feel your breathing and let go of everything else. Imagine a place that is special to you, where you love to be. It may be outside in nature, inside a house or from a picture or dream. Wherever it is go there now. Notice what it looks and smells like, see the textures and hear the sounds. In this special place, it is peaceful and beautiful. You feel safe and loved, happy and relaxed. You can feel your heart and known your own mind. You are free to be yourself and you decide who else can come in. You can invite someone you love to join you, or you can just be yourself. Whatever you choose enjoy some time for you in your special place.

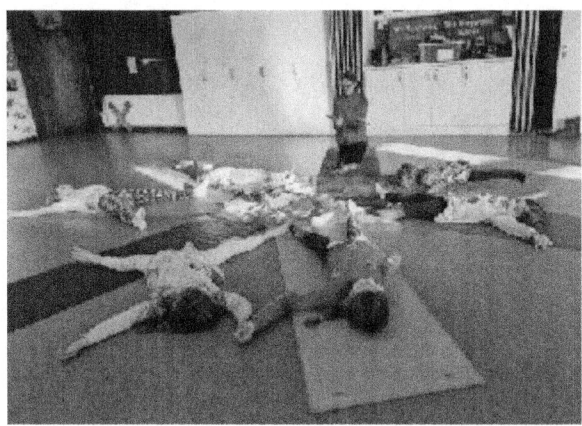

Tree Relaxation
Imagine yourself as a strong tree in the jungle, a forest, on a beach or in a city. Who do you shelter? What is the weather like? How do you grow and stay strong?

BEAUTIFUL ENDINGS

In India, Namaste, is a greeting in everyday life. In yoga it is a more profound gesture of respect towards another person.

Yoga traditionally beings with chanting. It can signify the start of the yoga class and a welcome to all. When chanting Namaste, the hands are put together in front of the chest or the third eye and bowing forward. It can be a time for the instructor to connect with all the students and make them feel part of the practise and that each student is valued.

Namaste translates to, I bow to you, or, the divine in me honours the divine in you. It is not meant to have a religious sentiment. It is a mantra of peace and equality to live by on and off of the yoga mat.

It is a lovely way to end the yoga session by chanting namaste together. It acknowledges that an instructor supports students and thanks students supporting them. It is a beautiful chant that connects people. It promotes the wonderful quality of non judgement of others and to always see the light in others, their light.

It represents that we are united, we are the same, we are one.

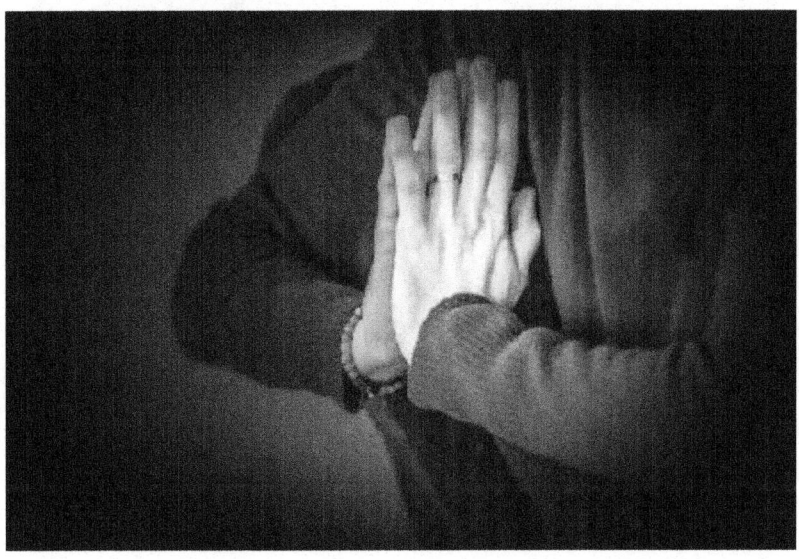

THE CREATIVE ACTIVITES

Craft activities that connect with the theme of the class have been a popular part of a yoga class with children. This activity is best completed at the end of the class. Reading a story to the children whilst they are working on their creations is a lovely addition to help deepen the connection of the theme of the class. There are suggested craft ideas in each lesson plan.

Drawing or colouring a mandala can help provide focus and relaxation for children.

A mandala is a spiritual symbol used by those in the Tibetan Buddhist Tradition. In Sanskrit, the language of Yoga, the mandala represents connection to life energy. The symbolism of the cycle of life is represented through the mandala. The exterior edge of the pattern represents attachments to the exterior world, relationships, expectations and attachments held in daily lives. The centre of the mandala represents the purest energy of life, free of all exterior world attachments.

Children may like to design their own mandalas by drawing or painting patterns, words, or objects such as a flower, which symbolises growth.

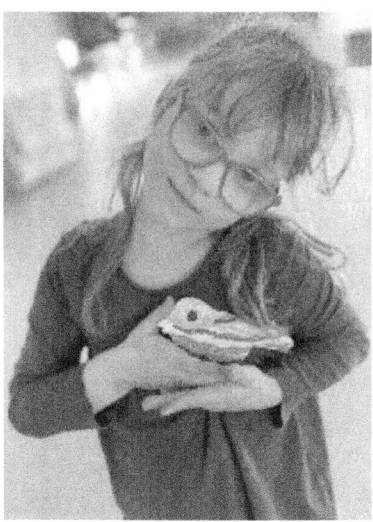
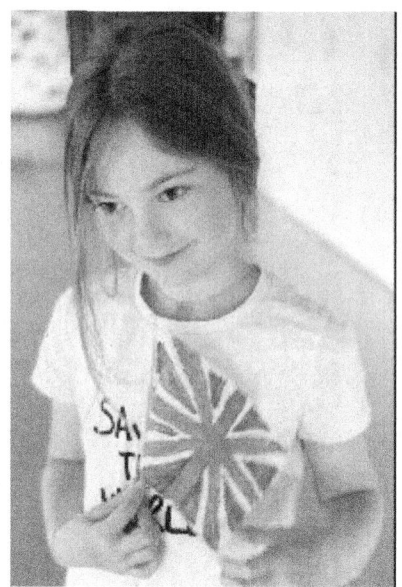

CHILDREN'S YOGA LESSON PLANS

BEAUTIFUL BUG BALL

INTRODUCTION
Today we will be going to a beautiful bug ball. Think about a bug / insect that you would like to be today at the ball. You can be the same bug as a friend or different, so many bugs are different from each other and all are welcome and beautiful just the way they are.

QUESTION TO CHILDREN
What is your favourite bug / insect?

BREATHING EXERCISE
Airwalk (Be a woodlouse on their back in this exercise)

WARM UP ACTIVITIES
Nature Kids - take turns to call out bugs / insects and move around the room in the way they do.

2 x Sun Salutations

ASANAS
Charades - using bug yoga cards or pictures.
Musical Mats - Beautiful bug ball

GROUP WORK
Dog Chase (using bugs, such as a spider chasing fly)

CRAFT - make a bug using clay, shells, beads and nature items

STORY - "How Beetle Got his Coat" from the book, "A World Full of Animal Stories by Angela McAllister.

BIRDS

INTRODUCTION
Birds are everywhere, you can see them in the garden, woods, towns, park and cities. Birds never stay the same, they change with the seasons and watching them can be super interesting. In spring you can look out for the first Swallow arriving from Africa, birds making their nests and baby birds hatching. If you get up early, you can hear their morning dawn chorus about an hour before it gets light. Robins, Blackbirds and Thrushes start the singing and many others join in. You can even be a bird detective, taking out your note book, binoculars and record what you see.

QUESTION TO CHILDREN
What is your favourite bird and why?

BREATHING EXERCISE
Bird Breath

WARM UP EXERCISES
Nature Kids. Think about how birds move, take turns to call different ways and copy movement, waddle, dive, fly, hop, shake feathers, run, glide…
Feather Race
2 x Sun Salutations

ASANAS
Practise different bird poses. Swan, Dove, Peacock, Owl, Eagle, Crow.
Make up your own pose to your favourite bird or a bird you like.
So many yoga poses are animals and many are birds. Connect with being the birds in the poses, maybe your arms become legs and feet or wings.

GROUP WORK
Rock, Tree, Bridge - birds perch on all three.
Bird Tunnel (Downward Facing Dog Tunnel)

RELAXATION
When birds sleep they often tuck their head under their wing or nestle their beak under their feathers. Find your most comfortable position to rest in.
Special Place

CRAFT - Bird Craft - colour a bird, draw your favourite bird, make a clay bird, paint a ceramic or wooden bird

STORY - "How the Swallows Tail Forked", Native American Story.
"Follow the Swallow" by Julia Donaldson

NIGHT TIME ANIMALS

INTRODUCTION
In our class today we are going to explore and connect with animals that are awake and active during the night, nocturnal animals. Animals that are awake in the day time are known as Diurnal animals.

QUESTION TO CHILDREN
What is your favourite nocturnal animal?

BREATHING EXERCISE
Lion Breath
Most lions hunt at night and are generally considered nocturnal animals

WARM UP ACTIVITIES
Nature Kids - Each child to take a turn to name nocturnal animals and leads the other children in how to move like them around the room.
2 x Moon Salutations

ASANAS
Night Time Animal Yoga Cards
Musical Mats

GROUP WORK
Bat Cave (Downward Facing Dog Tunnel)

RELAXATION
Animal Friend

STORY
"The Fox and the Star" by Coralie Bickford-Smith

CRAFT
Nocturnal themed animal craft.
Draw, colour, wooden craft or make from natural materials.

RAINFOREST ANIMALS

INTRODUCTION
Rainforest are wet and warm habitats. Trees grow very tall to compete with other plants for sunlight in the rainforest. There are Rainforests in Africa, Asia, Australia and North and South America. The biggest Rainforest is the Amazon Rainforest. Most Rainforests are found along the equator, where it tends to be hot. More than half of the worlds animals live in the Rainforest.

QUESTION TO CHILDREN
Can you think of any animals that live in the Rainforest?

BREATHING EXERCISE
Snake Breath

WARM UP ACTIVITIES
Nature Kids (Rainforest Animals) (Some of the animals of the Rainforests - varieties of monkey, jaguar, Birds of Paradise, sloth, frog, snakes, lemurs, ant eaters, river dolphins, fish, spiders)

ASANAS
Read the "The Kapok Tree" book by Lynne Cherry. Match or make up a pose for each animal in the book.

GROUP WORK
Tree Community- Trees are the lungs of our planet, they breath in carbon dioxide and breath out oxygen. Trees support each other under ground. We can be stable and strong when we support each other.

Make Nature Scenes - Rainforest

RELAXATION
Tree Relaxation

CRAFT - Sloth, draw, colour, decorate
STORY - "The Kapok Tree" by Lynne Cherry

BLOSSOMING

INTRODUCTION
The Earth around us is blossoming, we too can be like nature, blossoming to our full potential.
Just like the blossom tree that flowers when the earth nourishes it, in the same way we can nourish ourselves.
Yoga can help us to blossom and in our class today we will be exploring ways in which we can do that.

QUESTION TO CHILDREN
What helps you to feel like you are blossoming?

BREATHING EXERCISE
Alternate Nostril Breath
This breath can bring calm and balance to your mind.

WARM UP ACTIVITIES
Wheel Barrow Race - healthy play food
Clean living is part of a yogic lifestyle, the food we eat plays a large part of how we feel. Eating clean healthy foods not only feeds our physical body, it also invites us to connect with nature.
2 x Sun Salutations

ASANAS
Mantra Magic
Positive self talk is like magic, when we tell ourselves we can do something or are something we can become them.

PARTNER WORK
Partner Poses
Just like the blossom tree needs good soil, water, sun and air to blossom, so to our environment of family and friends can help us to blossom. Practise partner poses that lift and support each other.

RELAXATION
Loving Guided Meditation

CRAFT
Mandala draw or colour.

STORY
"How the Bear Clan Learnt to Heal". From "A Year Full of Stories" by Angela McAllister

CHRISTMAS YOGA PARTY

INTRODUCTION
Christmas is here once more. For many people it is a time to be with family having fun together, playing games, going for a walk and sharing food. For Christians it is the festival to celebrate the birth of Jesus.
Our class today is celebrating this holiday together in a fun Christmas themed yoga class.

QUESTION TO CHILDREN
What does Christmas mean to you?

BREATHING EXERCISE
Heart Mudra

WARM UP ACTIVITIES
Freeze Yoga Statues - Christmas theme, star, tree, reindeer, snowman…

ASANAS
Lucky Dip - Use this idea for Santas present sack, allow the children to pick a pose and then gift it to a friend. All children practise.
Musical Mats

GROUP WORK
Beachball Pass, pass the parcel, have a handmade gift for the children, stop music for each child to receive one.

RELAXATION
Guided Star or Inner Light

CRAFT - Using pine cones and mini felt balls, create a mini Christmas Tree

STORY - "The Snow Queen" by Hans Christian Andersen

EASTER

INTRODUCTION
Our class today is connecting with and celebrating the Christian festival of Easter. Do you know the Easter story? Good Friday marks the day that Jesus was crucified and Easter Monday celebrates Jesus rising again. Easter is also a time of fun and celebration for many families, celebrating the arrival of spring with fun time outdoors doing things like egg hunts and games.

QUESTION TO CHILDREN
What will you be doing to celebrate Easter?

BREATHING EXERCISE
Bunny Breath or Bee Breath

WARM UP ACTIVITIES
Easter Egg Hunt

ASANAS
Charades - Easter themed poses. Rabbit Pose, Boat Pose (nest), Lamb (Cat Pose), Frog Pose, Flower Pose, Butterfly Pose, Tree Pose.

GROUP WORK
Balance Asanas using an additional egg and spoon, or bean bags, add a garden games feel to the postures.

RELAXATION
Springtime

CRAFT - Draw, make, colour or decorate flowers, such as tulips or daffodils

STORY - "Basket of Eggs" from "A Year Full of Stories" by Angela McAllister

SPRING / SPRING EQUINOX

INTRODUCTION
The spring equinox is officially seen as the start of spring. It is a time to celebrate the joy of spring returning and the Earth blossoming once more. This special day is where there is a balance of light and dark, one of 2 days in the year when the day and night are equal in length. You may have noticed the days getting longer, flowers beginning to bloom, buds beginning to open on trees and plants and the air may seem warmer.

QUESTION TO CHILDREN
What do you like about spring?

BREATHING
All Good Things
Breathing can help to cleanse the lungs, helping to get rid of stale air and cleansing the body with new fresh air.

WARM UP ACTIVITIES
Feather Race
Migrating birds are returning with effortless grace, spring is a time for ease from their mental and physical flight.

2 x Sun Salutations
Celebrate the sun returning to warm the Northern Hemisphere (or the part of the earth where the children live) once more. Practise Sun Salutations with a sense of being thankful to the sun for its life giving energy.

ASANAS
Nature Yoga Cards
Connect with natures energy and beauty of spring through yoga postures. Tree Pose, Flying Bird Pose (Aeroplane Pose), Flower Pose for example.

GROUP WORK
Yoga Poetry or Group Yoga Pose Flow

RELAXATION
Springtime

CRAFT
Decorate a mini plant pot or glass and plant a bean seed

STORY
Greek Myth Persephone

MIDSUMMER CIRCUS PARTY

INTRODUCTION
In our class today we will be celebrating midsummer. Midsummer has the longest hours of daylight and the shortest hours of darkness. We will have a circus party in our gardens to celebrate.

QUESTION TO CHILDREN
What is your favourite thing about midsummer?

BREATHING EXERCISE
Airwalk. Children can pretend to be tightrope walkers

WARM UP ACTIVITIES
Hula Hoop challenge

ASANAS
Yogi Says (Ringmaster Says)

BALANCE WORK
Be an acrobat. Place a skipping rope on the floor or make a beam using yoga bricks. Ask the children to place a bean bag on their head, walk the rope or beam, jump off the end and hold a balance pose.

RELAXATION
Flower Garden

CRAFT - Make a Ringmasters Stick, decorate a stick

STORY - "The Elephant and the Blindman", from "A World Full of Animal Stories" by Angela McAllister

AUTUMN EQUINOX (MABON)

Mabon is a Pagan holiday that celebrates the autumn equinox in September in the Northern Hemisphere. This time of the year was celebrated in history all over the world. It was a time of celebration of the harvest season. Farmers know how well crops have done to ensure families had enough food for winter. It is and was a time for giving thanks for the harvest. It is a time of perfect balance when the hours of light and dark, day and night are equal. After the autumn equinox the nights will be longer than the days and a reminder that colder weather is not far away.

QUESTION TO CHILDREN
What are you thankful for this autumn?

BREATHING EXERCISE
Alternate Nostril Breath - Balancing and calming

WARM UP ACTIVITIES
Nature Kids
2 x Sun Salutations

ASANAS
Spin Game - Get ready for cosier nights together with family, reading and playing games together.

GROUP WORK
Plough Race
Partner Poses - representing the balance of the equinox

RELAXATION
Autumn

CRAFT - Decorate a special stick. Native American Talking Stick. This is a tradition of touring everyones voice. When a person holds the stick it is their turn to know that everyone is listening to what they have to say.

STORY - Native American Story

SAMHAIN (Sah-wen)

QUESTION TO CHILDREN
What does Halloween mean to you?

INTRODUCTION
In history an ancient festival marking the end of harvest season and beginning of winter was called Samhain. This festival has roots in being a pagan festival originating from Celtic tradition. Our ancestors believed that for one night the veil between the physical and spiritual world is at is thinest. Permitting the coming and going of loving ancestors spirits and even fairy folk. Halloween stems from Samhain.

BREATHING EXERCISE
Alternate Nostril Breath. Helps to calm the mind and find stillness.

WARM UP ACTIVITIES
Fairy Ring Dance
Some of our ancient ancestors believed that on Samhain you may even see the fairies dancing. Play Celtic music, The Fairy Reel is a great choice.

2 x Sun Salutations

ASANAS
Discover an Animal Friend

GROUP WORK
Trick or Treat. In history people impersonated their loved ones or ancestors spirits and visited houses, sharing a story about them and accepting offerings on their loved ones behalf.

RELAXATION
Guiding Star

CRAFT - Decorate a mask. Think about sharing your inner self in your mask.

STORY - A Celtic Mythology story, "The Women Behind the Door of the Moon" is a good choice.

VALENTINES DAY (LOVE) YOGA

INTRODUCTION
Our Yoga class today is one of connecting with our hearts. (This lesson plan can also be for Valentines day). We will be doing postures that connect with our hearts and also open this area in the body.

QUESTION TO CHILDREN
How big is your heart?, its about the size of your fist. What does the heart do? It pumps blood everywhere in the body. Recreate the beat of the heart together, using the fist gently beating against the centre of the chest. The heart beats around 100,000 times a day! What an amazing part of our body.

BREATHING EXERCIES
Heart Mudra

WARM UP EXERCISES
Love Train
2 x Sun Salutations

ASANAS
Mantra Magic - heart opening asanas

GROUP WORK
Yoga Poetry

Love it or Leave it

RELAXATION
Loving Guided Meditation

CRAFT - anything heart related, draw or colour a heart mandala

STORY - "Valentines Story" from "A Year Full of Stories" by Angela McAllister

WINTER

INTRODUCTION
Winter is a good time to slow down and recharge our energy. It is important for our health to change our energy and daily life with the seasons so that we feel as well and as energetic as we can. Just as nature changes throughout the year, we too can learn from her lead. Nature is still in winter, quieter and resting more. Many trees rest, animals hibernate and with longer nights we can sleep longer. We may spend more time indoors. In our class today we will be connecting with the energy of winter.

QUESTION TO CHILDREN
What is your favourite thing about winter?

BREATHING
Candle Breath

WARM UP ACTIVITIES
Freeze Yoga
Invigorating exercise each morning can help us keep well and fight off colds and flu.
2 x Sun Salutations

ASANAS
Twister

Group Work
Make Nature Scenes (winter)

RELAXATION
Radiant Star

CRAFT
Draw or colour a Robin

STORY
"Wee Robin Red Breast" from "A World Full of Winter Stories", by Angela McAllister

GARDEN PARTY

INTRODUCTION
The light of days are longer, warmer and we get to spend more time outside. We may have a garden to enjoy or a local park to play at. Today in our class we are going to celebrate this time of year with a garden party.

QUESTION TO CHILDREN
What is your favourite thing to do in the garden or park?

BREATHING EXERCISE
Bee Breath

WARM UP ACTIVITIES
Limbo
Under and Over

ASANAS
Yoga Assault Course - include yoga poses that relate to the garden such as Tree, Bird poses, Butterfly, Dragonfly, Worm (snake).

GROUP WORK
Cant Move Me - Connecting with the Earth

RELAXATION
Flower Garden

CRAFT - Flower Craft, make tissue paper flowers, draw or colour flowers, decorate a wooden flower

STORY - A Nature Story

SUMMER BEACH PARTY

INTRODUCTION
Summer is here. Summers energy brings fun and joy. Summers earth element is Fire. Fire is powerful. It warms, excites and fuels. Fire can inspire us to stand up for what we believe in and dance with life. In our class today we will have a beach party to connect with summers fun and joyous energy.

QUESTION TO CHILDREN
What is your favourite thing about summer?

BREATHING EXERCISE
Cooling Breath (Sheetali)

WARM UP ACTIVITIES
Limbo
2 x Sun Salutations

ASANAS
Beachball

GROUP WORK
Beachball pass

RELAXATION
Beach Relaxation

CRAFT - Paint a rock or shell

STORY - "How Jelly Fish Lost their Bones" by A Year Full of Animal Stories" by Angela McAllister

ANTARCTIC DAY

INTRODUCTION
Antartica, the coldest place on Earth. Antarctic Day marks the day of a treaty that was signed by countries around the world. The treaty prevents other countries from fighting over Antartica and ensures that every country has the freedom to explore and study it. Antartica is the 5th largest continent. Antartica is covered in ice yet many different animals species live there. Our class today will be connecting with this magical continent and finding out more about it.

QUESTION TO CHILDREN
Is there anything you know about Antartica that you can share with us? (Cold, continent covered in ice, home to 9000 different animal species, global warning is causing many icebergs to retreat and ice shelves to collapse. It is also warming the water which is having an affect on animals.

BREATHING EXERCISE
Lion Breath. Antartica is the coldest place on Earth, the temperature never gets beyond 15 degree celsius. Lion Breath can warm our body.

WARM UP ACTIVITIES
Icebergs. Antartica is covered in ice, ice bergs, glaciers and ice shelves. Ice shelves are floating masses of ice that has broken off from the main land.
2 x Sun Salutations. For 6 months of the year it is always daylight, the sun never sets in the summer, for the other 6 months of the year it is in darkness and the sun never rises.

ASANAS
Animal Yoga Cards or Animal Bags. There are 9000 different animal species that live in Antartica, such as birds, whales, seals, sea snails, penguins, sea cucumbers and algae.

GROUP WORK
Jammy Jazzing. Antarctic is quiet, there are no trees or plants to rustle in the breeze, no noise from traffic, people do not live there only scientist or people working. Start with silence and make your own entertainment.
Animal Chase - use animals such as an orca chasing a penguin

RELAXATION
Start Card - Can you imagine living in darkness for half of the year.

CRAFT - A Penguin story
STORY - Draw, colour, make or decorate a penguin.

HOLIDAY TO HAWAII

INTRODUCTION
We will be taking a trip Hawaii in our yoga class today. I invite you to imagine you are planning to go on this holiday, what sort of things will you want to pack? Hawaii is the largest of hundreds of volcanic islands in the Central Pacific Ocean. It is a tropical island so the temperature can be warm and breezy.

QUESTION TO CHILDREN
What will you pack for your trip to Hawaii?

BREATHING EXERCIE
Ocean Breath. This breathing exercise is a great way to soothe yourself wherever you are.

WARM UP ACTIVITIES
Hula Dance. Hula originated from the Polynesian people, the indigenous people of Hawaii. These people were voyagers and settled on the island of Hawaii. Over time the Hula has changed to add music and drum beats.

2 x Sun Salutations. The weather is warm all year around in Hawaii due to its close proximity to the equator.

ASANAS
Nature Yoga Asanas for Hawaii.
Volcano - Chair Pose, Flower Pose (flowers are in bloom all year, Hibiscus is national flower), Surfing - Warrior II, Palm Tree Pose - Tree Pose, Canoe - Boat Pose (Polynesian people used to visit other islands and fish), Shark Pose, Rock Pose, Dolphin Pose.

Surfboard Competition

PARTNER WORK
Partner Volcano

RELAXATION
Peace Relaxation

CRAFT - Make a Flower Lei. Draw or colour a Hibiscus Flower.

STORY - "A Hawaiian Story", "A Year Full of Stories" by Angela McAllister

BLACK HISTORY MONTH

INTRODUCTION
In the UK, Black History month is in October each year. This month is all about celebrating black people now and in history. This month started in the early 1900's as many black people were not celebrated or their stories shared. In our class today we will be celebrating black people and some of their stories of strength, courage and inspiring others to never give up.

QUESTION TO CHILDREN
Can you think of a person of colour that we can celebrate today?

BREATHING EXERCISE
Warrior Breath. Connecting with inner strength

WARM UP
Learn reggae basic steps and dance. Play One Love by Bob Marley. Bob Marley was from Jamaica who used his music as a way of raising a voice against oppression and to promote black pride

2 x Sun Salutations. Offer this salutations as an honour and respect for black lives

ASANAS
Share a story of an inspiring black hero or heroine. The story of Mary Seacole was shared in this class and poses matched to various parts of the story.

Warrior I - Mary was born in Jamaica around 200 years ago. Her mother was a nurse and a healer, her father a Scottish Soldier. As Mary grew up she worked with her mother and learnt about medicine and nursing. She looked after many sick people.

Aeroplane Pose - Mary loved to travel. In those days for a women and one who was mixed race to be allowed to travel was extremely rare. She visited England for 3 years and eventually married an English man. Mary was very brave, she returned to Jamaica in 1850 to nurse people with cholera and helped many people.

Gorilla Pose - In 1853 war broke out called The Crimean War. Mary went to the war office to request to join the Florence Nightingale Nurses to help treat soldiers but she was turned down.

Boat Pose - Together with a friend she decided she would go to help anyway. She opened a hotel in Crimea. It wasn't a hotel as we know today, it was a tin shack with food, supplies and somewhere for the soldiers to rest. Money made, Mary used towards medical supplies to treat soldiers who were, cold, hungry, injured and sick.

Bridge Pose - She built a bridge (metaphoric) so that soldiers could come to her and get help. She treated not only British soldiers but also Russian soldiers

Downward Facing Dog into Plank Pose - A lot of nurses did invaluable work looking after soldiers, but Mary went one step further. She rode on horse back into the battlefield to nurse injured men from both sides of the war. Soldiers called her, Mother Seacole.

Childs Pose - After the war she lead a quiet life living between London and Jamaica.

Candle Pose or Legs Up Pose - She received many medals for her bravery from Governments of different countries. She returned with little money and poor health. Soldiers wrote to newspapers and 80,000 people attended a charity gala for her to raise money. She lived out the rest of her life in peace.

QUESTION TO CHILDREN
What did they think about the story of Mary Seacole. What qualities did Mary have.

GROUP WORK
Gratitude Meditation

RELAXATION
Loving Guided Meditation

CRAFT - Explore black pride colours and paint or colour a rock or poster promoting black pride

STORY - Read an inspiring story of another black person in history

EARTH DAY

INTRODUCTION
More than a billion people around the world celebrate Earth Day. This days purpose is to raise awareness on protecting the planet from things like pollution and deforestation and ways to help look after the planet. Our class will be dedicated to this day and exploring ways we too can help keep our planet clean and safe for years to come.

QUESTION TO CHILDREN
What things do you already do, or what can you do to help look after the planet? (reduce waste, recycle, reuse, adopt animals, litter clean, use less water…)

BREATHING EXERCISE
Green Breath

WARM UP ACTIVITIES
Earth Missions
2 x Sun Salutations

ASANAS
Pop-stick Yoga with Earth Day themed poses

GROUP WORK
Gratitude Meditation
One of the best ways we can help look after the earth is simply to be content. We don't need everything. We can be happy with what we have. Having less stuff makes us happier.

RELAXATION
Special Place Card

CRAFT
Decorate a shell. Up cycle something old.

STORY
"Wangari's Trees of Peace" by Jeanette Winter.

INTERNATIONAL ANIMAL RIGHTS DAY (10TH DECEMBER)

INTRODUCTION

International Animal Rights Day shares the same date with Human Rights Day. The Human Rights Act started after World War II and since then campaigners have tried to have animals included in this act and day. It is campaigned that animals have the right to be treated with respect and acts of cruelty against them needs to end just as much as for humans. Around 25 years ago International Animal Rights Day began. This day is aimed to remember animals that have been victims of cruelty from humans and to persuade humans that kindness and respect is due to all sentient creatures. On this day thousands of animal rights supporters across the world hold candle vigils and other events to mark this day. Today we will hold our own vital in remembrance to animals and support kindness and respect to all beings. (Light a candle to burn during the class)

QUESTION TO CHILDREN
What is your favourite animal?

BREATHING EXERCISE
Lion Breath or Bear Breath

WARM UP ACTIVITIES
Nature Kids. How does your favourite animal move. Each child to take a turn.

2 x Sun Salutations. Dedicate the salutations to all animals that have suffered from humans

ASANAS
Animal Bag. Talk about the animals picked by the children. Can we do anything to help look after them.

PARTNER WORK
Time To Shine. Create a new yoga pose for your favourite animal and demonstrate to the rest of the group.

RELAXATION
Animal Friend

CHANTING
Om Shanti Shanti Shanti - Peace chant to send out into the world

CRAFT - make an animal, using clay, beads, feathers and any other crafts
STORY - A story about animals. "Animal Stories from Around the World" by Angela McAllister

INTERNATIONAL FRIENDSHIP DAY

INTRODUCTION
International Friendship day is a great opportunity to celebrate friendships and we will be doing just that in our class today. What qualities make a good friend? Open discussion about qualities - kind, supportive, understanding, patient, flexible, generous, loving, trusting, a good listener. Its also important to be a good friend to yourself as well as to others so that when we treat ourselves in these same ways we feel good.

QUESTION TO CHILDREN
What do friendships mean to you?

BREATHING EXERCISE
Heart Mudra

WARM UP ACTIVITIES
Circle of Friends
Synchronised Sun Salutations - working together can give us strength and union.

ASANAS
Yoga Jenga

GROUP WORK
Partner Poses

Community Circle

RELAXATION
Animal Friend

CRAFT - Make a friendship bracelet

STORY - "Androcles and the Lion" Aesop Fable

INTERNATIONAL PEACE DAY

INTRODUCTION
International Peace Day is a global holiday celebrated yearly on the 21st September. This day was started in 1981 by the United Nations. Peace Day asks us to commit to peace above all differences and to help build a culture of peace. We will dedicate our Yoga class today to world peace. (Light a candle to represent support for world peace).

QUESTION TO CHILDREN
What does peace mean to you?

CHANTING
Om Shanti x 3. Peace chant.

BREATHING EXERCISE
Peace Breath. We can bring peace to the world each day by a little meditation.

WARM UP ACTIVITIES
Over and Under. Cooperation is part of us and is a principle of peace learning. If cooperation was the single most dominant behaviour at all levels of society, the whole human world would be a step closer to world peace.
2 x Sun Salutations. Pause at end of salutations with hands in prayer at heart as a symbol of peace.

ASANAS
"I am Peace" by Susan Verde. Read book and do poses and affirmations given in book.
Book includes group work.

RELAXATION
Peace Relaxation

CRAFT - Draw or colour the peace sign, or a dove the animal that represents peace

STORY - "A Story of Peace" from "A Year Full of Stories" by Angela McAllister

WORLD BEE DAY

INTRODUCTION
World Bee Day (20th May) is a global day to raise awareness of the importance of bees and other pollinating animals and the threat that they face from human impact.
Do you know 90% of wild flowers and 75% of food crops depend entirely on bees and other pollinators.
World Bee Day aims to help protect bees and pollinators by raising awareness on how to look after them.
Individually we can do things to help bees.

QUESTION TO CHILDREN
Can you think of any ways to help bees and pollinators?
(plant native plants that flower during different parts of the year, make bee houses, leave water out in the garden, buy bee friendly products, buy raw honey from local farmers, buy products from sustainable farming).

BREATHING EXERCISE
Bee Breath

WARM UP
Pollinators Game
2 x Sun Salutations

ASANAS
"Are you A Bee", book by Judy Allen, or similar book about bees and pollinators. Read book and practise poses that match the story.

GROUP WORK
Female bees do a dance when they find flowers to let their sisters know where the flowers are. Working in small groups fly together to find flowers, then create a bee dance to show your sisters. Perform bee dance to the other children.

RELAXATION
Rainbow Flower Garden

CRAFT - Draw or colour a bee. Paint a wooden bee decoration. Make a seed bomb using clay and wild flower seeds.
STORY - "Saint Patrick and the Bees", from "A World Full of Animal Stories" by Angela McAllister

WORLD HEALTH DAY (7th April)

World Health day is celebrated on the 7th April by countries all over the world. This day is dedicated to promoting benefits of good health and well being for all and that everyone should be able to access health essentials.

QUESTION TO CHILDREN
Can you think of things we can do to have good health and well being? Discuss healthy living with the children.

BREATHING EXERCISE
Easy Breath

WARM UP ACTIVITIES
Yoga Pretzels
Celebrate our bodies and what they can do
2 x Sun Salutations

ASANAS
Yoga Spin Game
Connecting with others can bring feelings of happiness and wellness

GROUP WORK
Plough Race
Inversions can help to balance the system, calm the nervous system and turn things upside down

RELAX
All is Well

CRAFT
Mindful colouring cards or picture

STORY
"How the Bear Clan Learnt to Heal", "A Year Full of Stories" by Angela McAllister

WORLD MUSIC DAY

INTRODUCTION
In our Yoga class today we will be celebrating music from around the world. World Music Day is all about celebrating the greatness of music and the gift it brings to our lives and the world. (Play music from around the world, Puto Mayo's "Music from Around the World for Children" is a fantastic choice).

QUESTION TO CHILDREN
What is your favourite style of music or song?

BREATHING EXERCISE
Didgeridoo Breath. The Digereridoo is a wind instrument that originated with the Indigenous people of Australia, the Aboriginal people of Northern Australia. This instrument can play low sounds and holds a beat. When playing its a bit like breathing exercises in yoga, controlling your breath. (Play music from Australia). (Music from the continent of Australia)

WARM UP ACTIVITIES
Jump the Mats. (Play music from Africa).
2 x Sun Salutations. Play music from India, "Pi's Lullaby" is a good option. (Music from the continent of Asia)

ASANAS
Olympic Games Yoga Assault Course. The Ancient Greeks invented the Olympic Games. In history these games held a music and instrument competition. Play Greek music. (Music from the continent of Europe)

GROUP WORK
Rock Tree Bridge. Rainforest music celebrated the beauty of nature. Play music of South America. (Music from South America)

Jazzy Jamming. In the Antarctic there is silence, no trees for the wind to rustle. There may be sounds of ice cracking. Explorers and scientists would bring their own music for entertainment.

RELAXATION
Special Place

CRAFT - make a musical instrument, use shells and sticks, or bells and sticks

STORY - "The Song of the Armadillo", from "A World Full of Animal Stories" by Angela McAllister

WORLD OCEANS DAY

INTRODUCTION
World Oceans Day is a wonderful opportunity to celebrate our oceans of the world and their importance in our lives. It's also an opportunity to think about how we can help to look after our oceans.

QUESTION TO CHILDREN
Are there things you are already doing to help look after the oceans?
or
Can you think of any ways we can help to look after the oceans?

BREATHING EXERCISE
Oceans Breath

WARM UP ACTIVITY
Beach Volley Ball
2 x Sun Salutations - 60% of our body is water. When this energy flows well in our body this water can nourish and cleanse us just as water does in nature when it is flowing. Connect with flowing in the salutations.

ASANAS
Put on Diving Gear

GROUP WORK
Make a group kelp forest
Make a group coral reef

RELAXATION
Beach Relaxation

CRAFT - Decorate shells
STORY - "The Mermaid of the Magdalens" from "A Year Full of Stories" by Angela McAllister

WORLD WATER DAY

INTRODUCTION
World Water Day is a yearly International Day held on the 22nd March. This global day aims to highlight the importance and value of water and to be grateful for how lucky we are to have clean safe water.

Many people's access to clean water is threatened by pollution, growing population, agriculture and climate change. There has been some great work, 90% of the Worlds population now have access to improved sources of drinking water, however still much work needs to be done. World Water Day aims to have clean water sanitation for all.

QUESTION TO CHILDREN
What does water mean to you? (how important is water to you, your family, home and life)

BREATHING EXERCISE
Ocean Breath or Rainbow Breath

WARM UP ACTIVITIES
How can we help preserve water? (Lessen time in the shower, turn of the tap when brushing teeth, take own water bottle out with us, spread the message of saving water, harvest rain water.
Go With the Flow - Don't waste water assault course

Two Sun Salutation sequences

ASANAS
Put on Diving Gear
Water provides life to all living things. Explore animals that live in water

GROUP WORK
Pick a selection of the yoga poses practised and allow the children to create a flow. Play music and flow through the sequence of poses.

Wash Away

RELAXATION
Be a Rainbow

CRAFT - Rainbow activity, colour wooden beads and make a rainbow keychain
STORY - "The Little Raindrop" tells a story of the water cycle. World Water Day Story.

WORLD WILDLIFE DAY (ENDANGERED ANIMALS)

INTRODUCTION
World Wildlife Day, 3rd May, is a Global day that gives opportunity to celebrate the many beautiful wild plants and wild animals that we share the planet with. It is also a day to raise awareness of the dangers that threaten the survival of many animals in the world. Critically Endangered these are animals that are at extremely high risk of extinction. Endangered, are animals facing a very high risk of extinction. Vulnerable, are animals that are considered to be facing a high risk. Animals can become extinct through deforestation, pollution, hunting and human impact. This can feel overwhelming, however there are things that we can do to help.

QUESTION TO CHILDREN
Can you think of any ways that you can help animals that face or are already endangered? (Learn about animals in danger, plant trees, recycle, reduce waste, use natural products, work together to clean up habitats, look after animals in your area, adopt animals that are at risk, support environmental causes such as No Deforestation and World Wildlife Fund.

BREATHING EXERCISE
Elephant Breath. The African Forest Elephant is currently Critically Endangered due to them being hunted for their ivory.

WARM UP ACTIVITIES
Iceburgs / habitats. When areas become smaller they can only support so many animals for food, water, shelter and safe places to raise their young.
2 x Sun Salutations

ASANAS
"Endangered Animals" book by Rachel Hudson or similar. This book has rhyming poems about the animals that the children can then guess what the animal is. Match or make up a pose for each animal.
Option - establish what animals are currently listed as endangered and print off some pictures, learn a little about the animals to share with the children then either match a yoga pose or invite the children to create their own.

GROUP WORK
Yoga Poetry

RELAXATION
Animal Friend

CRAFT - Draw or colour one of the animals.
STORY - African Folk Tales have some wonderful animals stories.

SELF ESTEEM

INTRODUCTION
Self esteem is how a person feels about themselves. Most of us will have dips in self esteem as we go through different stages or challenges in life. When we have good self esteem we may feel confident, have a positive image of ourselves and are willing to try new things. When we have negative self esteem we may lack confidence, put ourselves down and avoid new things. Yoga practises can help us to build our self esteem. We will explore some of these in the class today.

QUESTION TO CHILDREN
Share something that you like about yourself?

BREATHING EXERCISE
All Good Things. The way we talk to ourselves has a lot to do with how we feel, when we fill ourselves with positive thoughts we feel and become them.

WARM UP ACTIVITIES
Partner Mash Up
According to Yoga philosophy, we are all connected. When we work together it feels good.
2 x Sun Salutations

ASANAS
Mantra Magic & Positive Affirmations
Do you ever have thoughts that you can't do something, or you aren't good enough at something? We can challenge these negative thoughts about ourselves. We can question what we would say to a friend if they told us the thoughts. Treating yourself as if you were a friend can really help to change negative self talk to kind talk about ourselves.
Balance Poses
Discuss that its ok to fall, or make mistakes, its how we learn, everybody makes them. If we keep practising we will be able to do challenging things.

GROUP WORK
Make a structure. Everybody is needed for their part to make the structure.

RELAXATION
Positive Thoughts

STORY - "Why Wisdom is Everywhere" from "Wisdom Tales" by Heather Forest
CRAFT - Draw a self portrait to remind yourself how wonderful you are

GRATEFULNESS

INTRODUCTION
Sometimes we can be bombarded with adverts that can leave us feeling unsatisfied. Gratitude means being thankful for what we already have in our lives. When we are grateful our bodies release chemicals that make us happier and calmer. Even in the most down moments we can find something to be grateful for.

QUESTION TO CHILDREN
What are you grateful for?

BREATHING EXERCISE
Back to Back

WARM UP ACTIVITIES
Friendship Circle - Grateful for friends
Or
Yoga Pretzels - Thankful for amazing bodies
2 x Sun Salutations - grateful for the life giving energy from the sun

ASANAS
Grateful Asanas
Musical Mats

GROUP WORK
Group Massage

RELAXATION
Guiding Star

CRAFT
Decorate a glass jar. Write or draw post it notes with something we are grateful for. The children can take them away and write or draw one each day putting them inside.

STORY
"The Dog and his Reflection" Aesop Fable

HAPPINESS

INTRODUCTION
Happiness is unlimited and contagious and sharing ones happiness with others can bring a lot joy in others peoples lives. In the class today we will be celebrating happiness.

QUESTION TO CHILDREN
What makes you feel happy?

BREATHING EXERCISE
All Good Things

WARM UP ACTIVITIES
Human Knot
2 x Sun Salutations

ASANAS
Animal Bag
Animals bring a lot of joy and love
Musical Mats

PARTNER WORK
Partner Poses
Connecting and supporting others can bring feelings of happiness.

RELAXATION
All is Well

CRAFT
Paint or write a positive message on a rock, leave it for someone.

STORY
A happy story of your choice

KINDNESS

INTRODUCTION
Yoga philosophy believes in practising kindness everyday. This philosophy believes that kindness begins with the mind and our thoughts. That we should talk kindly to ourselves even if a mean comment comes up, we can learn to observe these thoughts and find ways to think about ourselves differently. Kind self talk helps us to develop kind thoughts and words about ourselves and others. It begins with ourselves and it is said that we should talk to ourselves as we would a friend.

QUESTION TO CHILDREN
What does kindness mean to you?

BREATHING EXERCISE
All Good Things - practising positive self talk

WARM UP EXERCISES
Human Knot. Be kind to each other in this game, patient, gentle, supportive

2 x Sun Salutations. Practise kindness with yourself, being gentle, listen to your body, respecting your limits, notice how you feel.

ASANAS
Mantra Magic. Practise the power of kind and positive self talk.

PARTNER WORK
Partner Poses. Practise kindness and support of each other.

RELAXATION
Loving Kindness Relaxation

CRAFT - Postive Mantra on a rock

STORY - "Lion and Mouse", Aesop Fable

MINDFULNESS

INTRODUCTION
To be mindful is to be aware of what is happening right now. Being mindful can help us to calm our thoughts and emotions. It can help us to feel more peaceful, no matter what is happening around us. In our class today we will be practising ways to be mindful, its a bit like having some magic tricks that you can do to help calm or focus yourself.

QUESTION TO CHILDREN
Do you have any things you already do to help you feel calm and peaceful?

BREATHING EXERCISE
Easy Breath. Focusing on your breath is one of the best magic tricks to calm your mind and help you to be in the moment, in a peaceful state.

WARM UP ACTIVITIES
Emotional Exploration
Being mindful with your emotions is another magic trick that can help you to understand them and let them go from your mind and body. Sometimes we can hold tension in our bodies, show example, invite the children to stand up and pretend to feel tense and stressed, discussed what happens to their body, did they tense their body in any areas? Practise Emotional Exploration warm up activity.

ASANAS
Discover an Animal Friend.
Animals are experts at being mindful and in the moment enjoying themselves with what is happening in the now. Invite the children to spend some time outside of the yoga class to watch animals to see if you can observe this.

GROUP WORK
Mirroring. Another magic trick to be mindful and find a peaceful calm is meditation. We will be trying a mediation with a partner known as mirroring.

RELAXATION
Positive Thoughts

CRAFT - Colour or draw a mandala. Make a mindfulness bag, draw or write mindful magic tricks learnt and place them in a bag. When you need to be mindful take one from your bag to help you.

STORY - Mindfulness story for children, suggestion - "The Three Questions" by Leo Tolstoy.

MY AMAZING BODY

INTRODUCTION
Today we are going to be celebrating our amazing bodies. It's really important to look after them inside and out with healthy food, exercise and positive thoughts about our bodies. Practising Yoga can help us to be kind and loving to our body. Take a moment to think about how you feel about your body.

QUESTION TO CHILDREN
Can you think of ways to help look after your body?

BREATHING EXERCISE
Air Walk - Connecting the breath and movement of the body

WARM UP EXERCISES
Yoga Pretzels
2 x Sun Salutations - moving slowly and gently being kind to the body

ASANAS
Operation - connecting with how postures can promote health in different parts of the body
Time to Shine - celebrate the amazing things the body can do

GROUP WORK
Partner Poses

RELAXATION
Body Awareness

CRAFT - Decorate a picture frame to remind yourself how amazing you are. Draw a self portrait.

STORY - An inspiring story, such as a story from "I Am Not a Label" by Cerrie Burnell.

MY AMAZING IMAGINATION

INTRODUCTION
Today we will be celebrating our amazing imaginations. A very famous scientist said, "Imagination will take you everywhere, Imagination embraces the entire world, giving birth to evolution". Imaginations are limitless. Great imaginations write beautiful poetry and stories, or are used to create new inventions. We will be connecting with ours in our class today.

QUESTION TO CHILDREN
How do you use your imaginations? I use mine to help me create Yoga classes.

BREATHING EXERCISE
Rainbow Breath

WARM UP ACTIVITIES
Catch a Butterfly
Yoga Limbo

ASANAS
Magical Yoga Stories

GROUP WORK
Rainbow Power Partner

RELAXATION
Special Place Card

CRAFT - Make a rainbow coloured bracelet or keyring using wooden beads.

STORY - Read a magical tale such as "East of the Sun West of the Moon" by Brooks Bowman

LOVE YOGA

INTRODUCTION
Yoga is an ancient practice that originated in India some 5000 years ago. Drawings on clay have been found of people sitting in a cross leg position to suggest people practised yoga in ancient times. The ultimate aim of yoga is to calm the mind from busy thoughts so that we unite with the peaceful feeling within. Yoga can bring so many benefits, physical strength and flexibility, it can help us to calm the mind from busy thoughts, it can help us to balance our inner health systems and also to experience inner contentment.

QUESTION TO CHILDREN
What is your favourite thing about yoga?

BREATHING EXERCISE
Balloon Breath

WARM UP ACTIVITIES
Yoga Limbo
2 x Sun Salutations

ASANAS
Memory Yoga Game

GROUP WORK
Group Yoga Flow

RELAXATION
Colour Meditation

CRAFT - Draw or colour a mandala

STORY - An Indian mythology story of one of the asanas

SHINE YOUR LIGHT

INTRODUCTION
Some of the months over winter can have longer hours of darkness than light. When its dark outside we can bring light inside our homes. (Question to children). Another way is to connect with our inner light, our inner selves and make our lights shine bright. In our class today we are going to look at ways to keep our inner lights shining brightly.

QUESTION TO CHILDREN
Can you think of any ways to bring light inside. (candles, fire, cosy lights)

BREATHING EXERCISE
Candle Breath. This breath can help to calm the mind and help us to connect with our inner light.

WARM UP ACTIVITY
Firefly Dance. Light is essential to live, all energy comes from the sun. Animals relate to light in different ways. Rooster crows at sunlight, a baby turtle will use light to find the ocean, fireflies make their own light. How do you feel when you stand in the sun?
2 x Sun Salutations - the darker days will pass and the longer lighter days will return.

ASANAS
Mantra Magic Asanas
We can charge our inner lights to shine brighter by celebrating our qualities and identify what things we do well at. Think about something that you are good at or you do well at. Create a mantra or affirmation to go with your quality, for example, "I am kind and giving". Chose a pose to match your mantra and practise whilst repeating your mantra, notice how you feel.

GROUP WORK
Yoga Flow with poses practised. Once our lights shine brighter we can take them out into the world to shine for others.

MEDITATION
Candle Meditation

RELAXATION
Inner Light

CRAFT - Make some white clay tea light holders and once dry allow the children to paint, colour and decorate.
STORY - "Legend of the Poinsettia" by Tomie dePaola

CHINESE NEW YEAR

INTRODUCTION
(date) is the start of the Chinese New Year. This is the most important holiday in China. The celebrations start with a new moon that happens between the end of January and February. The celebrations lasts for 15 days until the next full moon. It is a time to honour household and heavenly as well as ancestors. Its a time for family, being together and feasting.

QUESTION TO CHILDREN
Is there anything you already know about Chinese New Year?

BREATHING EXERCISE
Dragons Breath. The dragon is a symbol of China, it symbolises wisdom, power and wealth and is believed to bring good luck to people.

WARM UP ACTIVITIES
Tai Chi - learn some basic Tai Chi and share it with the children. This ancient Chinese tradition evolved into a gentle and mediative exercise.
2 x Moon Salutations.

ASANAS
The Chinese Calendar. This calendar includes the Chinese zodiac, a cycle of 12 signs that align with the path of the sun through the universe. Each Chinese New Year is marked by one of the zodiac signs which are animals. This year is the year of the (animal). Match Yoga Poses to the 12 animals. Goat, Horse, Dragon, Tiger, Rabbit, Monkey, Snake, Rat, Dog, Boar, Rooster, Ox. Practise the poses

GROUP WORK
Lantern Parade. After 15 days, celebrations end with a lantern parade. Children go out at night carrying lanterns, the lantern symbolises people letting go of the past and looking to new beginnings. Walk around the room in a parade, carrying a tea light if possible, play traditional Chinese music, when the music stops hold a zodiac animal pose of your choice to show in the parade. Continue until a natural end.

RELAXATION
Lantern Meditation

CRAFT - make a paper Chinese lantern

STORY - "Chinese New Year Story" from "A Year Full of Stories" by Angela McAllister.

DIWALI

INTRODUCTION
Diwali is about good triumphing over evil. It is a celebration of hope, happiness and peace. Diwali is celebrated by millions of people around the world. Hindu', Sikh, Jain and other religions come together for five days to celebrate this festival of light. The festival originated in India and marks the beginning of a new year that coincides with the Hindu calendar. We will be connecting with Diwali and finding out more about what happens during this festival.

QUESTION TO CHILDREN
Is there anything you know about Diwali you can share?

BREATHING EXERCISE
Candle Breath - Diwali is known as the Festival of Light. Millions of people light small oil lamps and place them in houses, gardens, roofs and more.

WARM UP ACTIVITIES
Don't wake the Dragon (Demon). Diwali has a famous legend where Prince Rama and his wife Sita return after they defeated an evil demon.
2 x Sun Salutations - light candles in the middle of the room to represent the festival of light

ASANAS
Provide a selection of yoga cards that are relevant to Diwali and share information. River Pose - The River Ganges in Indian, Hindus believe the river is holy. Goddess Pose - Hindus worship many gods and goddesses, Lakshmi is a goddess honoured at Diwali and is asked to drive away misfortune. Temple Pose - Hindus worship at home and at temples during Diwali, where offerings of food, flowers and prayers are done. Flower Pose - people draw rangoli patterns on the floor outside their homes during Diwali to invite gods into their homes. Candle Pose - representing the Festival of Light.
Musical Mats with poses learnt, play music for Diwali

GROUP WORK
Make structures - rangoli pattern, temple, festival of light scene

RELAXATION
Inner Light

CRAFT - Rangoli Patterns, draw, colour, decorate
STORY - "Rama & Sita the Diwali Story" from "A Year Full of Stories" by Angela McAllisteer

HARRY POTTER YOGA

INTRODUCTION
Have you read any of the books, watched the films or heard of Harry Potter? If you haven't, Harry Potter is a wizard who attends a school called Hogworts. The stories are all about Harry and his friends attending the school and their adventures in learning magic and defeating dark magic.

QUESTION TO THE CHILDREN
Who is your favourite Harry Potter character and why?

WARM UP ACTIVITIES
Love Train - (Hogworts train to Hogworts). Once arrive at Hogworts sort children into Gryffindor House. Courage, bravery and determination, these are the traits of Gryffindor House, the bravest house at Hogworts.

BREATHING EXERCISE
Lion Breath - The house crest of Gryffindor has bold colours of red and gold represented by a roaring lion.

WARM UP ACTIVITIES
Quidditch - Over and Under add an additional hoop for the teams to throw their ball (golden snitch) through at the end. Determination is needed.

ASANAS
Cat Pose, Owl Pose, Toad Pose (Frog), Rat (Childs/Mouse)
Each student at Gryffindor receives their own pet. Practise the poses and each student chooses which pose they will have. After 1,2,3 the children take the pose of the pet they chose.

Charm Lesson - Lumos Spell (light). Remote control tea lights work well for this. Give each child a wand (stick). All children to take Wizard Pose (Warrior 2) and point their sticks to the centre. After 1,2,3 the children say Lumos making the lights alight.
Winguardian Leviosa Spell (levitation). Half the children be students, half the children prepare for Crow Pose. After 1,2,3 the children say Winguardian Leviosa and the children fly into Crow Pose. Swap over.

PARTNER WORK
Herbology - look after a magical plant. Working in partners, one child becomes a seed in Childs Pose, their partner helps to nurture them so that they can grow into a magical plant. Invite the children to be creative and ask what their plant is. Ensure each child gets a go to grow into a magical plant.

Broomstick Flying - Musical mats with poses practised in the class.

CHALLENGE POSE
Defence Against the Dark Arts. Choose a challenging asana to practise. A posture that needs courage to defeat the dark magic of Voldemort.

RELAXATION
Astronomy Class - Guided Star

CRAFT - Decorate a wand, a stick and natural craft materials create a wand
STORY - choose a extract from the first Harry Potter book, "The Philosophers Stone" by JK Rowling

OLYMPIC GAMES

INTRODUCTION
(date) is the start of the Olympic Games in (location). These games started in Ancient Greece some 3000 years ago. The games have become one of the worlds prestigious sporting competitions for many elite athletes. We will be holding our own mini olympic games in our class today.

QUESTION TO CHILDREN
Will you be watching any of the games, if so what are you looking forward to seeing?

BREATHING EXERCISE
Warrior Breath. Connect with your inner power

WARM UP ACTIVITIES
Pass the Torch. The Olympic Flame is a symbol of connection between ancient and modern games. Several months before the games a torch is lit in Olympic, Greece. The ceremony starts with a torch relay which ends with lighting the Olympic Cauldron during the opening of the games and burns for the duration of them.

2 Surya Namaskar

ASANAS
Yoga Assault Course. Time to be an yoga athlete

CHALLENGE POSE
Handstand. Takes determination and practise to be an athlete

RELAXATION
Rest and relax your athlete's body on the mat you deserve it.

CRAFT - make a gymnastics ribbon using a stick and ribbon

STORY - Read a story of a Paralympian

Printed in Great Britain
by Amazon